Getting Better

Getting Better

A Doctor's Story of Resilience, Recovery, and Renewal

ANDREW GABOR KADAR, MD

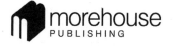

The content of this book is for informational purposes only and is not intended to diagnose, treat, cure, or prevent any condition or disease. This book details the author's personal experiences and opinions and does not constitute health or medical advice. This book is not intended as a substitute for consultation with a licensed practitioner. Please consult with your own physician or healthcare specialist about your personal healthcare.

The publisher and the author are providing this book and its contents on an "as is" basis and make no representations or warranties of any kind with respect to this book or its contents. The publisher and the author disclaim all such representations and warranties as permitted by applicable law, including but not limited to warranties of healthcare for a particular purpose. In addition, the publisher and the author assume no responsibility for errors, inaccuracies, omissions, or any other inconsistencies herein.

In order to protect their privacy, some people's names have been changed in this text.

Morehouse Publishing, 19 East 34th Street, New York, NY 10016

Morehouse Publishing is an imprint of Church Publishing Incorporated.

Cover design by Emily Weigel
Typeset by Nord Compo

A record of this book is available from the Library of Congress.

ISBN 978-1-64065-705-2 (hardcover)
ISBN 978-1-64065-706-9 (ebook)

To the doctors, nurses,
and staff of Cedars-Sinai Medical Center,
especially those who took care of me.

And to my family:
Rachel, Kenny, Kelsee, and Christine.

Contents

Part III
Home Recovery

Part IV
Recovery to Renewal

Preface

> Everyone who is born holds dual citizenship, in the kingdom of the well and in the kingdom of the sick. Although we all prefer to use only the good passport, sooner or later each of us is obliged, at least for a spell, to identify ourselves as citizens of that other place.
>
> —Susan Sontag, *Illness as Metaphor*

S everal years ago, I faced a sudden, unexpected illness that required treatment with open-heart surgery. As I recuperated from my operation, I wanted to make sense of what was happening to me. Reflecting on the physical and mental challenges generated by my illness and recovery, I realized that writing about these events, viewed through my dual perspective as both a patient and a doctor, could benefit others as well.

My initial concept was to describe the experience of heart surgery, confining the narrative and discussion to cardiovascular disease. However, all severe illnesses share common elements. Therefore, much of what I observed could be helpful for people facing any type of medical crisis. Each patient's experience is unique with its own specific course of healing, but the pattern of forward progress interrupted by setbacks is shared by everyone who suffers and recuperates from a major illness. And since these events affect family and friends, my narrative is designed to inform an even larger circle of readers and help them navigate through a medical storm.

The jiujitsu prospect of producing something helpful and positive out of the maelstrom of a dreaded predicament motivated me to write this book.

PART I

DENIAL, ACCEPTANCE,
AND RESILIENCE

Chapter 1

Recognizing the Unseen:
The Subtlety of Symptoms

Everything is funny as long as it is happening
to somebody else.

—Will Rogers

Chest pain—should you worry? How about a headache or abdominal pain? Are these fleeting symptoms of little significance or the first signs of a deadly disease? Each of us needs to decide when life throws us such a curve. You don't want to ignore a warning of something severe. You also don't want to be a hypochondriac. What do you do? Call a doctor right away? Brush it off as insignificant? Wait to see if the pain recurs? The right response isn't always obvious. And even when it should be obvious, we may not want to see what we dread.

What happens when a perfectly healthy person, or somebody with the self-image of being such a healthy person, feels a worrisome symptom?

- It could be abdominal pain: Indigestion? Appendicitis? Obstructed bowel? Kidney stone? Or any one of multiple other causes? Entire books have been written on the variety of causes for abdominal pain.

- Headache: Probably tension but could it be increased pressure from bleeding inside the skull or a brain tumor?
- Chest pain with exercise: Muscle strain, acid reflux, or heart disease? Could be heart disease but for a person with no prior history of heart disease, how hard is it to write it off as a muscle strain or something else that will go away on its own?

Symptoms can come and go. When you feel fine, that episode of chest pain, or any other pain, can be rationalized. You may think, *No big deal. It didn't hurt that much, and now it doesn't hurt at all.* If it happens again and then a third time, it may be harder to ignore, but denial can persist.

The flip side of denial is seeing doom in every symptom. Not all chest pain is a heart attack, and every headache doesn't signal a brain tumor. As a matter of fact, most chest pain is not due to heart disease and the vast majority of headaches don't have deadly causes.

All of us must perform a balancing act between excessive worry, vigilance, and denial. Modern medicine performs miracles—cures otherwise deadly diseases and prolongs life. But you usually have to get to a doctor first. When serious illness strikes, early intervention can save the day and delay may be deadly.

Having medical knowledge can make your balancing act easier, but denial is powerful. When you're too close to a patient, judgment can suffer. There is a good reason why surgeons generally don't operate on their immediate family members. Emotions get in the way when a medical decision is about you or a loved one.

My own transition from a doctor to a patient gave me new insight into the denial and fear patients feel. I also got a taste of the frustrations, both small and large, that patients experience during the course of their hospitalization and recuperation. But take heart, it's not all gloomy. The triumphs on the road to recovery, also small and large, produced joy along the way. This is a hopeful story.

Just days after Halloween, I found myself in the hallway leading to the cardiac operating rooms at Cedars-Sinai Medical Center, where I'd been working for many years as an anesthesiologist.

What was unusual was that instead of doing my job in a comfortable set of teal-green scrubs, this time I was feeling utterly vulnerable and a bit ridiculous in nothing but a flimsy, open-back exam gown. Instead of comforting and sedating a patient—taking care of another person whose life is in peril—I was on the receiving end of an IV, flat on my back on a gurney as my colleagues rolled me down the long corridor to the OR.

Even before the first dose of sedative began to numb my brain, the whole experience seemed utterly unreal. I'd evidently been cast in some bizarre drama as an exceptionally healthy man about to undergo open-heart surgery. Strangely, my predominant emotion was not fear but amazement mixed with a sprinkling of outrage. My inner voice was screaming, *This should not be happening to me!*

Of course, lots of people have protested, "I was so healthy before this!" but it's a futile lament. As a physician, I was well aware that disease often strikes unexpectedly and indiscriminately. You don't have an illness—or at least you don't know you have it—until the day it shocks you with pain, hemorrhage, paralysis, or some other nasty symptom.

I knew that, but I still couldn't help feeling betrayed by my body. My predicament made no sense: I didn't develop severe coronary disease because of bad habits. I got it despite having done everything right.

I'd not neglected my health; I had consistently maintained a health-promoting lifestyle. Just a few days earlier I would surely have been high on the list of those least likely among my contemporaries to suffer from heart disease. I had always checked out on the favorable side of nearly every cardiac risk factor.

Habits: nonsmoker.

Weight: always close to the insurance-table ideal.

Blood pressure: on the low side—if anything, better than normal.

Diabetes: no.

Family history: excellent.

A past history of elevated blood cholesterol on long-ago lab tests was the only chink in my otherwise sterling heart-health profile. After I started on medication, my cholesterol level came down and had stayed normal for over seven years by this time.

In fact, I had never suffered from any major medical problems of any kind. Unlike many of my young buddies who'd fractured arms and legs, I'd gone through a boisterous boyhood without breaking a single bone. I'd competed as a gymnast for my high school and university, specializing in pommel horse and rings. In a fitness test during my freshman year at UCLA, I did 107 push-ups in one minute and was still going strong when the time was up. Being athletic and fit had been a vital part of my self-image ever since. I worked out regularly with exercise machines and weights. I hiked, ran 10Ks, and frequently climbed up four flights of stairs to avoid waiting for an elevator.

My father had lived to be 94 and had trekked in the Canadian Rockies at 86. Though my mother had passed away from cancer at 77, she'd never had heart problems. Even my maternal grandfather, born in the nineteenth century, lived into his late eighties.

With both good habits and good heredity, there was no apparent reason for me to have heart disease. All I could think was, *This must be a horrible mistake.* I may have conveniently disregarded my unavoidable risk factors— being male and 62 years old—because I felt so much younger.

Just before his death, Pulitzer Prize–winning writer William Saroyan quipped, "Everybody has got to die, but I have always believed an exception would be made in my case." My delusions hadn't extended quite that far, but despite continuing to encounter desperately sick people in my work, I'd never given any thought to the possibility of suffering a serious illness myself. I was fully convinced that wouldn't happen for at least several decades.

There is never a good time to be ambushed by heart disease—or any other dreadful illness, for that matter— but just three months after my wedding? That was horrible-nasty-bad timing. Rachel, my wife, thought I was a paragon of good health. As she watched me being wheeled toward an uncertain fate, I wondered if she was having any second thoughts, any regrets about coupling her future with mine.

Despite her being quite a bit younger than me, Rachel had sometimes struggled to keep up with my energy level, even asking for time-out to rest. Suddenly the tables were turned, and I needed a major time-out. Lightning had struck, and the amount of damage done was yet uncertain. Rachel was surely shell-shocked. We both were. This was definitely not the life we had expected to share. Like it is for many patients, our future suddenly had a new element: uncertainty.

As my gurney rolled away from my new wife, I looked back and saw my usually vivacious bride holding back tears. I couldn't help but feel regret tinged with guilt for bringing all this down on her. As a doctor, I had seen this before, but now it was really hitting home: illness doesn't just afflict the patient; it's a family affair.

Ten days before being taken into surgery for that triple coronary artery bypass, I had been working out in the gym of my condo building while watching the 6:00 p.m. *PBS NewsHour*. I'd been working out in that gym regularly, three to five times a week. Since no one but the building's residents were permitted to exercise there, and only a few ever did, it was almost like having my own personal health club.

That evening I'd started gliding on the elliptical machine, as usual, gradually increasing my speed. Nine minutes into a 20-minute run, at near-sprint velocity on a 30-degree incline, I suddenly felt a burning sensation in my chest, under the sternum.

Hmmm . . . Probably heartburn.

But I knew what heartburn felt like, and this felt different. I stopped exercising, and the pain ceased right away.

Gosh. What's going on?

The possibility that this could be a symptom of heart disease flashed across my mind. How could it not? Most people know that chest pain can be the first sign of a heart attack. Besides, I was a doctor who treated heart patients all the time. I knew well that exercise-induced chest pain, located under the sternum, and relieved promptly by rest—precisely those three elements—made up the classic textbook triad of the most common presentation of coronary artery disease, the underlying cause of heart attacks.

Cholesterol, calcium, and other substances in the blood can cling to the inside of blood vessels, a process called *atherosclerosis*. Over time, such deposits can increase and eventually interfere with normal blood flow. When that happens in the arteries that supply the heart, it is called *coronary artery disease*, or *CAD* for short, the most prevalent heart malady around the world.

But I was equally aware that many other conditions can produce chest pain. Anything that irritates the esophagus can cause it—most commonly acid reflux (heartburn), but also esophageal muscle problems that impair the proper movement of food into the stomach. Other sources of chest pain from the digestive system includes stomach ulcers, gallstones, and pancreatitis. Inflammation of the lining of the lungs (*pleuritis*) can produce a sharp pain with every breath, and especially with a cough or sneeze. Problems with the lungs, such as pneumonia and pulmonary hypertension, can result in chest pain. Anxiety can also be a trigger.

Among athletes, simple muscle strain is a common cause. I was no stranger to chest-muscle pain, having encountered it numerous times from strenuous workouts and foolishly sustained injuries, both during my years competing in gymnastics and after. The worst occurred during high school, when I partially tore some muscles while working on a new gymnastics move.

The pain during my condo gym workout didn't *feel* like a muscle strain, but I was so sure I didn't have heart disease that I quickly concluded that the burning sensation in my chest was a minor strain caused by an inadvertent move, a one-time event of no significance. Nevertheless, I ended my workout.

No sense in continuing when I don't feel well.

Having decided that the pain was insignificant, I didn't say anything about it to Rachel, either.

Why worry her over nothing?

Three days later, again around nine minutes into a vigorous elliptical workout, the burning returned. I stopped gliding, and the pain went away. After a couple of minutes of rest, standing on the machine and drinking three gulps of water, I resumed exercising.

The burning started again, this time after less than two minutes.

What the hell is going on?

The pain wasn't particularly severe, maybe a three on a scale of ten. Apprehension, far more than the burning itself, made me step off the machine and sit on a bench.

I don't have heart disease. This can't be angina.

(*Angina pectoris*: chest pain caused by inadequate circulation to the heart.)

Those were my reflexive thoughts again, but I continued to evaluate the situation.

Okay, I definitely feel burning in my chest, but it's not very strong. No other symptoms. No pain radiating to my left arm or chin. It's just in the center of my chest, under the sternum. I don't feel any pressure on my chest, certainly no "elephant standing on it"—not even a mouse. No excessive sweating or shortness of breath. No dizziness or lightheadedness.

I placed my left index and middle fingers on the thumb side of my right wrist to feel my radial pulse.

Strong and regular. No arrhythmia. No problem here.

The chest pain ended quickly. After just a few seconds on the bench I felt fine, as if nothing had happened. But something *had* happened . . . not just once but three times. I had experienced repeated episodes of exercise-induced chest pain relieved quickly by rest.

If somebody else had reported this symptom history to me, I would have recommended a prompt cardiac workup, starting with an electrocardiogram and a treadmill stress test—the former to detect heart compromise at rest and the latter with exercise. But I still believed that coronary artery disease was highly unlikely for me.

When I returned upstairs, Rachel remarked, "That was a short workout."

"I wasn't feeling good, so I stopped."

"Are you okay?"

"I'm fine."

Rachel stared at me intently with wide-open eyes. She had been concerned about my health since the previous month.

We had traveled to Taiwan for her brother's wedding reception. That's where Rachel was born and where the rest of her family lived. On two occasions while there I'd felt dizzy after touring several hours, albeit in 90-degree weather with 90 percent humidity. Once, when we were hiking at a hillside village celebrated for its expansive, misty vistas, I sat down on a bench for a few minutes until the feeling went away.

Three days later in Taipei, inside the cavernous, octagonal Chiang Kai-shek Memorial Hall, Rachel and I watched the changing of the guard in front of the nearly 33-foot-high bronze statue of the seated generalissimo. The soldiers went through an elaborate ten-minute routine—stepping, saluting, and rotating rifles in choreographed, near-robotic unison.

Right after the marching stopped, I shuffled with much less precision to a corner of the hall. I felt woozy and lay down on the floor. I knew that by placing my head no higher than my heart, I could prevent fainting and possible injury from a fall. After a few minutes, the lightheadedness passed.

I'd blamed both episodes on heat and dehydration, which can certainly cause dizziness, but Rachel hadn't been convinced. She had urged me to have a medical evaluation upon our return home. I didn't see any urgency: just a situation easily explained and quickly resolved. I could recall similar episodes of dizziness with heat and dehydration at least twice in the past, the first nearly thirty years earlier.

Following our return to Los Angeles, I worked out in the gym with 20-plus minutes of aerobics followed by 10 to 15 minutes on weight machines more than a dozen times without problems, prior to my first episode of chest pain.

Rachel asked me again to get a medical evaluation after my second troublesome workout. This time I told her, "I'll make an appointment. I'm due for a checkup anyway."

The next day I called my internist's office and was told that the earliest available appointment would be eighteen days away. Since office schedulers are neither trained in nor expected to gauge medical urgency and make triage decisions, they tend to prioritize appointments on a simple first-come-first-serve basis. A wait that long might have been okay for a routine visit, but I realized that my symptoms called for a prompt evaluation, so I asked to talk directly to the person who could make such an assessment: my doctor.

With his full head of gray hair and calming voice, Dr. Kevin Drury, my internist, rates high on the warm-and-fuzzy scale. He is renowned for taking all the time necessary to explain health issues to his patients, never making them feel rushed. Patients put up with long delays in his office because they know that once they get to see him, they'll receive personalized, high-quality care.

Kevin happens to specialize in cardiology, a fortunate coincidence given my complaint. After I told him about my chest pain, he seemed surprised but not alarmed. He scheduled me for a stress test on the following Tuesday.

My symptoms must have sounded suspicious enough to investigate but not so urgent that the workup couldn't wait five days. I asked myself, had I downplayed anything? Had I described events in a way that made them sound less ominous? I wasn't sure, but despite hoping for the best, I wondered if I should have asked Kevin to see me sooner.

But it was already Thursday afternoon, and my situation wasn't a genuine emergency. I felt fine at that moment. Kevin no doubt had a full schedule of patients already booked for Friday, and his office was closed during the weekend. I figured that if Tuesday was more convenient for him than Monday, waiting five days instead of four was unlikely to make any difference.

After the phone call, I told myself, *It'll probably be nothing, just a fluke, something benign. If he's not alarmed, I shouldn't worry, either.*

Had the patient been somebody else, the most likely diagnosis would have been obvious to me. But this wasn't anyone else, and my self-image—my identity as a paragon of good health and fitness—was on the line. No matter how classic my symptoms seemed, I just wasn't prepared to view myself as a heart patient, so I rationalized myself out of any urgency I was feeling. Aside from my doctor, I hadn't told anyone else about my symptoms. In particular, I hadn't said anything else to Rachel.

No sense in raising her anxiety level for nothing.

Rachel had come from Taiwan to the United States alone at age 26 to study English at California State University, Fullerton. Within a couple of years, while continuing her studies, she became fluent enough to conduct bilingual office work for a language institute. She later became an American citizen and switched to a career in real estate. With a vivacious personality and a strong work ethic, Rachel built her client list to become a successful agent.

Rachel was a bundle of effervescence. I was smitten from the start with her lovely face, brilliant smile, and lush black hair that cascaded way past her shoulders. She projected charm, charisma, and enough chutzpah to get away with some audacious behavior. For instance, during her first months working in real estate, she had canvassed for clients by passing out flyers and business cards in a neighborhood near her office. One day a woman confronted her, complaining, "Enough already! You real estate agents are driving me nuts, constantly harassing me. I wish all of you would just go away and leave me alone."

"Okay, I will," Rachel responded, flashing a mischievous smile. "But look at me. I'm so cute! How can you get mad at me?"

Both the woman and Rachel simultaneously burst out laughing. "Honey, that's the best line I've heard in a long time," the woman told her.

With the ice broken, she took Rachel's card, and they engaged in an extended friendly chat, getting to know and like each other. That woman, Karen, later introduced Rachel to several friends who were interested in either buying or selling a house. Rachel and Karen stayed in contact, and the story of their initial meeting became legendary in my wife's real estate office.

After making the appointment with my doctor for testing, I went to work on Friday. No problems occurred.

On Saturday UCLA played Arizona at the Rose Bowl, preceded by the annual Varsity Club tailgate party. Rachel and I went with another couple, the husband a former UCLA gymnastics teammate of mine and a lifelong friend.

We arrived hours before the game but still had to park at a distant fairway of the golf course that served as the stadium parking lot. We trekked a mile over grass fields and concrete walkways to the tailgate tent. Shortly before kickoff, we hiked to the stadium and up a legion of stairs to seats near midfield.

During the game, I was so engrossed in the action that I didn't even think about my recent episodes of chest pain. In the final two minutes, an Arizona field goal clinched the visitors' 29–21 victory. Afterward, we meandered across the golf course and back to our car.

I felt no discomfort throughout any of this. Whatever may have caused me pain during the strenuous workouts on the elliptical didn't appear to be interfering with any of my other usual activities. That reinforced my hope and bolstered my belief that nothing perilous was threatening my health. I pushed aside the knowledge that people with CAD often went about their daily lives without any symptoms until the moment they suffered a fatal heart attack.

Jim Fixx helped launch a fitness movement with the 1977 publication of *The Complete Book of Running*. It remained on the bestseller list for more than a year and inspired countless people to discover the joys of jogging. The author became a star, a celebrated evangelist for the health benefits of his sport.

Although he'd once been a two-packs-a-day smoker and overweight, Fixx had turned his life around when he began running. For seven years following the publication of his book, Fixx extolled the virtues of exercise for better health and longevity. He ran ten miles a day, played tennis, and engaged in other aerobic activities. He wrote additional books and articles on the subject and lectured to large audiences.

On July 20, 1984, at the age of just 52, Jim Fixx collapsed by the side of the road during his daily run and died on the spot from a massive heart attack. His autopsy revealed that one coronary artery was 95 percent blocked, a second 85 percent, and a third 70 percent.

According to his former wife, Mr. Fixx had suffered no prior symptoms; he never had any warning.

"If he did," Alice Fixx said, "he ignored it."

Between one quarter and one half of the people who suddenly drop dead from heart disease are said to have had no prior symptoms.[1] That adds up to around a 100,000 to over 200,000 deaths[2] each year of Americans who didn't even know they had heart disease. A forewarning of chest pain (or less commonly shortness of breath, nausea, or excessive sweating) can be lifesaving. If heeded.

Six months before Fixx died, while researching an article about a famous Boston Marathon runner, he had visited a clinic directed by Dr. Kenneth Cooper, another exercise guru. Cooper invited him to undergo a treadmill stress test that could have detected electrocardiogram abnormalities and led to preventative intervention.

Fixx declined.

The day after the football game was October 31. Rachel and I had made plans to go to the West Hollywood Carnaval, an over-the-top Halloween street festival. With several hundred thousand people expected to attend, parking anywhere nearby would have required getting there before dawn.

We decided to arrive after the party was in full swing. At 7:00 p.m. we met another couple at a restaurant about ten blocks from the event. After a light meal, the four of us began walking toward Santa Monica Boulevard, the site of the festivities.

I was decked out for the occasion in lederhosen and a gray Alpine hiking hat, topped with a jaunty white feather, souvenirs of a trip to the Austrian Alps. Rachel was simply dressed as herself, in jeans and a long-sleeved gray T-shirt.

I'd always had a natural tendency to walk faster than most people and usually had to hold myself back when strolling with others. That night, however, we were less than halfway to Santa Monica Boulevard when the burning sensation in my chest returned. I slowed down, causing us to fall farther and farther behind our friends.

As I struggled to decide whether to continue or stop, Rachel slowed beside me. Perhaps she thought I was taking my time to observe the colorfully costumed revelers around us. Torn between denying I had a health problem and the fear of harming myself by neglecting it, I tried walking ever slower. But even as I steadily decreased my pace to a near crawl, the pain kept getting worse. I knew that if this actually was angina, and I pushed on, I could precipitate a heart attack.

My growing anxiety finally overcame my pride.

"Rachel, I'm . . . not feeling well. I need to stop and rest."

"What's the matter, honey?"

"Not sure . . . just feel a little pain in my chest."

We were then outside a funky pizza-and-pasta place with a bench in front for customers waiting for a table. I sank down on the seat as Rachel stared at me, her brow furrowed.

On our recent vacation in Italy, I had easily climbed what the guidebook stated were 463 steps to the magnificent dome of the cathedral of Florence. During our long walks throughout that trip, Rachel had often asked me to slow down or stop for her to rest. This time I rested while she ran ahead to explain to our puzzled friends that I wasn't feeling well . . . perhaps from the meal we had just eaten.

When she returned, Rachel asked, "Do you want to go home? We don't need to go to this."

Though she might have preferred to leave, I insisted, "I'll be okay. Just need a little rest."

What was I thinking? Had this been some other guy, I would have told him to go straight to the Cedars-Sinai Emergency Room, only a few blocks away.

I sat and watched the crowd. Batman and Robin strolled by, then Gumby holding hands with a cowboy. Another young man ambled past us, laughing and chatting with his companions, a wooden knife handle drenched in fake blood protruding from the center of his chest.

My chest looked normal but was hurting for real.

Beside the burning ache around my breastbone, I had no other symptoms—no shortness of breath, no sweating, no dizziness. After a couple of minutes, the pain ceased, and we resumed walking slowly toward Santa Monica Boulevard.

We passed a sidewalk vendor cooking bacon-wrapped hot dogs. They smelled delicious and were selling briskly, hot off the grill. I walked past the stand, as far away from it as the sidewalk would allow, trying to get beyond its enticing aroma, fearing irrationally that even fumes of cholesterol might threaten my well-being. The situation felt eerily like a scene out of a movie, such as the James

Bond film *Live and Let Die*, in which a throng of revelers joyfully laugh and dance in a Mardi Gras procession, unaware that something ghastly is taking place in their midst.

When we reached the boulevard, I tried to enjoy the celebration, taking in the sights and shooting photos of some of the more colorful characters.

Rachel kept scrutinizing me and asking if I was okay. Our apprehension made it difficult for either of us to enjoy the spectacle, so we left for home after only an hour. Walking very slowly, we plodded the ten blocks back to the car, where I dropped into the driver's seat with relief.

On Monday I went to work as usual. I took elevators instead of stairs and otherwise limited my physical activity to avoid another episode. The day passed without a problem.

Cedars-Sinai Medical Center has operating and recovery rooms on multiple floors. My job required overseeing an array of operations and diagnostic procedures, some of which took only minutes, others many hours. On any given day I might administer anesthesia for a simple hernia repair, a complex and bloody abdominal aortic aneurysm resection, or the delicate excision of a brain tumor. The variety and range of cases offered a stimulating mix of challenges. So did providing comfort, reassurance, and TLC—tender, loving care—to my patients and their loved ones before and after procedures.

Anesthesiology requires being on your feet much of the time and performing tasks such as placing breathing tubes in windpipes and catheters in hearts. On Tuesday I finished a short schedule of cases before noon. Since my treadmill test was not set to begin until 4:30 p.m., rather than wait around the hospital I drove the three miles home with plans to eat lunch and rest.

When I arrived at our condo, Rachel was on a business phone call at her desk. Happy to see me home unexpectedly early on a weekday, she said goodbye to her client, bounced out of her seat, hugged and kissed me, then pulled me toward our bedroom. Given my health concerns, I hesitated at first, but not for long.

Then in the middle of everything, the burning chest pain reappeared. Once again, now with even more ambivalence and distress, I felt torn between admitting I had a health problem and risking a heart attack. My pride, desire, and fear of death were grappling in mortal combat. I'd heard gossip and jokes and read medical reports of men suffering heart attacks during sexual activity. People had snickered about Nelson Rockefeller allegedly dying that way, and an article in *New York* magazine had reported the wisecrack that he "thought he was coming, but he was going." Never before had I considered that as even a remote danger for me.

As the humorist Will Rogers noted, "Everything is funny as long as it is happening to somebody else." Things are not nearly so laughable when they're happening to you.

As I rolled onto my back, my anxiety began to ease as the pain ceased; however, my sense of relief was only partial and guarded. Having suffered yet another episode of the classic pattern of symptoms, I had even more reason to fear the likely cause.

For the first time, I felt death lurking just outside my field of vision.

Chapter 2

That Pivotal Moment:
When Tests Reveal a New Reality

> Life is what happens to you while you're busy
> making other plans.
>
> —John Lennon

If you seek medical care, your doctor is obliged to take a history—listen to your complaint and ask questions about your prior medical problems. It takes time and costs money. A physical exam can be uncomfortable (a medical euphemism for pain). "Does it hurt if I push here?" Every diagnostic procedure ordered—whether it's drawing a blood sample, taking a chest X-ray, doing a colonoscopy, or performing a heart catheterization—carries a risk. An old saying declares, "If you do something for a cold, it will go away in a week. If you don't, it'll last seven days."

People sometimes go to doctors for trivial reasons, but my situation was ominous. Ignoring it would have been foolhardy. I began by denying the obvious, rationalizing, and searching for a benign explanation, but I made an appointment with my doctor just days after my first episode of chest pain.

In a few heartbeats, I went from full-time doctor to full-time patient.

A doctor's life is not easy. The hours are long; you sometimes work all night. I've joked in the past that patients are very inconsiderate. They get sick at all hours of the day and night, and then expect you to take care of them, no matter how inconvenient the timing is for their doctors. Of course, nobody (okay, almost nobody) chooses to get sick, and doctors make a voluntary choice to train for their profession. I wouldn't say medical students know what they are getting into, because there are plenty of surprises along the way. You don't really know what a job entails until you do it. Working as a doctor also produces stress. Your patients' lives depend on your performance. For an anesthesiologist, that's true every time you administer drugs that keep people from feeling pain during surgery but can also kill. All of that is outweighed by the satisfaction of being able to alleviate pain, to help cure disease. Being a doctor, earning the trust of people to attend to their health, is a profound privilege. Hardly anybody thinks being a patient is a privilege.

I arrived at Dr. Drury's office, relieved to be on my way to a definitive diagnosis. Wearing hospital-issued teal scrubs, I entered the treadmill test area. The nurse asked me to lie down on the examining table.

The nurse attached conducting pads (electrodes) to my chest and recorded a 12-lead electrocardiogram (ECG). With each beat, an electrical impulse (generated by specialized cardiac cells, not the ECG machine) moves through our hearts, causing the chambers to contract in sequence.

As this wave travels from one section of cardiac muscle to the next, the electrocardiogram records the electrical activity, displaying it as a tracing of voltage over time.

ECGs are done to look for rhythm disturbances and signs of cell damage due to inadequate blood circulation to the heart muscle. Our hearts pump blood throughout our bodies, but to do so they need a steady supply of blood—and the oxygen and nutrients within it. Damage to cardiac cells disrupts the usual movement of positively charged atoms (sodium, potassium, and calcium) across their cell membranes. This leads to deviations from the normal electrocardiogram pattern. By recording changes in voltage over time between different pairs of electrodes, a standard 12-lead electrocardiogram allows doctors to identify areas of the heart with abnormal electrical activity and pinpoint the location of damaged tissue.

An electrocardiogram tracing begins at a baseline, the level of electrical potential across cell membranes just before the start of a heartbeat. The first small blip, called the *P wave*, heralds the contraction of the upper collecting chambers of the heart. In a normal pattern, the heart returns to baseline until a larger blip, the *QRS wave*, signals contraction of the ventricles, the lower chambers, and again returns to baseline. The pattern concludes with a third blip, the *T wave*, marking the relaxation of the ventricles. When a section of the heart fails to receive an adequate supply of oxygen-carrying blood, the tracing between the end of the QRS and start of the T wave either rises above or dips below the baseline. This is called an *ST elevation or depression*. Its size correlates with the severity of circulatory insufficiency. The different tracings in the 12-lead ECG allow doctors to identify the portions of the heart affected.

The pattern of my resting ECG looked normal and revealed no ST deviations or any other abnormal patterns. It was just like all the other routine ECGs in my chart from previous years. I felt somewhat reassured by this evidence that my heart showed no sign of having suffered an injury.

The nurse instructed me to walk two steps over to the treadmill, taking care that all my wires remained firmly attached.

Dressed in a traditional long white doctor's coat, Dr. Kevin Drury entered the room. I started walking on the treadmill to record my electrocardiogram during exercise. Two minutes and forty seconds into the test, with the pace far slower than my usual pace in the gym, the burning sensation in my chest began. I told Kevin. He immediately shut off the treadmill.

"I'm ending this test *now*," he declared, with unfamiliar urgency in his voice and firm emphasis on the final word.

I glanced over at my electrocardiogram and sucked in a breath.

Wow, that's one sick-looking ECG, I thought. *That can't be me!*

My ECG showed large ST depressions in nearly all 12 leads, a sign of severe circulatory insufficiency to most of my heart. It looked like the ECG of a man having a massive heart attack, except as I stood there, staring thunderstruck, the still-running recording slowly regressed to a normal pattern.

The pain from walking on the treadmill promptly ceased, but seeing the tracing made me feel much worse. In a daze, I stepped off the track. Still tethered to the ECG

machine by a dozen wires, I staggered backward a couple
of steps and sat down on the examining table for support.
My worst fear was confirmed. A thin film of tears formed
over my eyes, blurring my vision.

My normal resting ECG, both before and after the conclusion of the stress test, reassured me. I had not suffered
irreversible heart damage, meaning that I did not have a
heart attack. But my ever-decreasing exercise tolerance,
the chest pain, and the ECG tracings presented a dire picture. There was no denying it any longer. *Damn it! I have
coronary artery disease.* The next time I felt burning in my
chest, it could be the start of a heart attack.

I had no further illusions about my diagnosis. The stress
test proved that *atherosclerotic plaques,* fat deposits inside the
walls of at least one of my coronary arteries, had decreased
that artery's inner diameter by enough to keep a portion of
my heart from getting an adequate amount of oxygen-rich
blood. My normal resting electrocardiogram, along with
the fact that I had no symptoms at rest, indicated that my
coronaries remained sufficiently open to supply the blood
that my heart needed to beat at a rate appropriate for light
activity. But when the demand for oxygen increased with
exercise and my heart needed to beat faster, my coronary
arteries could not keep up. Insufficient blood flow to the
heart muscle then produced chest pain.

Kevin made some comment about this possibly being
something other than coronary artery disease. I figured
he said that only to try to make me feel better. He'd
stopped the treadmill test prematurely because he'd seen
enough. Continuing any longer could have precipitated
a heart attack and the need for immediate hospitalization
with emergency intervention. It could also have led to

my death, right in his office. Clearly bad for everyone involved.

In real life, unlike on TV medical shows, symptoms usually mean what they usually mean. A well-known adage in medicine states, "When you hear hoofbeats, don't think of zebras." A diagnostic workup, like a detective investigation, starts with an examination of the most likely suspect. My presentation—chest pain with the ECG changes brought on by exercise—looked, walked, and quacked like coronary artery disease.

This condition can continue to evolve slowly, with the vessels narrowing over months and years, progressively decreasing the patient's ability to exercise. That's exactly the process that had to have been going on for me for years already, as layer after layer of fat and calcium deposits—called plaque—silently and secretly clung to the inside walls of my coronary arteries, until at least one of the channels became narrow enough to cause angina and finally get my attention.

The larger the plaque in the coronary arteries grows, the more likely that a portion of the buildup will become unstable and crack. Just as a clot forms over a cut or an abrasion, one can develop over an injured section inside an artery. This can suddenly close off the artery completely. Alternatively, a piece of plaque can break off and float along an artery until it lodges in a narrower portion of the vessel downstream. This process can also completely cut off blood supply to part of the heart. Without circulation, heart cells die, an event we call a *myocardial infarction*, or more commonly, a heart attack.

Medical science has not yet discovered a way to predict which pattern my heart would follow, slow or sudden.

Nevertheless, the bad and even worse possibilities left me feeling stunned and deflated.

At this point in time, we knew my diagnosis but still didn't know the extent of the narrowing in my coronary arteries. An X-ray study called a *coronary angiogram* provides that information. Kevin got on the phone to schedule me for the study. My stress test performance called for urgency but didn't indicate an emergency, which meant that further workup should proceed within days but not necessarily right away. Since it was already late afternoon, Kevin scheduled my angiography for the following day.

My procedure was a late add-on to the schedule. It would take place sometime in the afternoon, after other patients' previously scheduled examinations were completed. If the doctor ended up doing an angioplasty, an X-ray-directed procedure to open up a partially blocked artery, I would have to stay overnight and miss work the next day.

After the angioplasty, I would have to take a blood thinner daily for several months. That meant a greater risk of bruising and bleeding, especially with trauma. *I am not playing tackle football and rarely get a bruise,* I tried to reassure myself. I could go on with my normal activities, except for having to be more careful about bumping into doors or slipping and falling. *Not a big deal.* Except my situation in its entirety was a very big deal. I felt crushed by the sobering and depressing realization that I had become a heart patient. My prior self-image as an unusually healthy specimen was shattered.

Fear and denial were waging a tug of war in my mind. *My heart is a ticking time bomb with a fuse of unknown length . . . Nah, I'll be fine. Kevin would have admitted me to the hospital if the danger was that high. I'll just take it easy until tomorrow afternoon.*

I left Kevin's office with prescriptions for metoprolol (a beta blocker) and nitroglycerine. The beta blocker was to lower my blood pressure and heart rate. Fewer heart beats against less pressure resistance translates to a lower energy requirement, reducing the chance of damage to the heart from too little oxygen for its workload. Nitroglycerine dilates coronary arteries, allowing more blood to supply all portions of the heart.

Kevin instructed me to take metoprolol right away, along with an aspirin to "thin" my blood, to make it less likely for a clot to form inside a blood vessel. The nitroglycerine would serve as my rescue medication. I would take that only if I had chest pain.

On my way home, I stopped at a CVS pharmacy. This time, instead of walking up the flight of stairs from the parking lot to the store, I waited for the elevator. I even took the elevator to go down. I had good reason to be apprehensive. Many people have paid a high price for ignorance or denial.

"So how did it go, honey?" Rachel asked as soon as I got home.

"Not as good as I'd hoped. I need to have another test tomorrow, an angiogram. They need to look more closely at the blood supply to my heart with X-rays. I may have to stay in the hospital tomorrow night."

Rachel stared at me intently, her brown eyes on the verge of tears.

"Is it dangerous?" she asked, her voice trembling.

I tried to reassure her.

"Not very. They do a lot of these at Cedars. Nearly everybody goes home feeling better the following day."

Rachel's expression relaxed. I told her the test would probably take place in the afternoon, after I finished my cases. She had previously planned to work at her office in Arcadia, around a half-hour drive each way. She decided to still go there in the morning but return in time to be at the hospital during my angiogram. She later told me that from the way I described the study, it didn't sound ominous, just something that could be tucked into our schedules after completing the day's work. I wasn't consciously downplaying the seriousness of the situation, but my attempt to keep her from worrying apparently had that effect. In retrospect, without meaning to mislead her, I did.

A little later, I called the Anesthesiology Department scheduler to let him know I probably wouldn't be available for cases on Thursday, the day after my angiography.

"Are you sure you want to work tomorrow?" he asked. "We can cover for you if you don't feel well."

I was scheduled to perform procedures in one of my favorite locations in the hospital. I am usually reluctant to give up those cases. Perhaps I was also on autopilot, expecting to work and disregarding the gravity of my situation. Doctors often work while sick. The profession instills an obligation to fulfill your responsibilities, take care of your patients, show no weakness, prove you're made of iron. One anesthesiologist I know worked until the week she delivered her baby and was back in the operating room three days later.

I assured our scheduler that I felt well enough to complete my lineup the next day. That didn't turn out to be the most prescient answer. I had trouble getting to sleep and woke up feeling apprehensive, too preoccupied with my own health to concentrate fully on the health of others. After all, I was about to have a procedure on my own heart. An angiography is usually quite safe, but catastrophes do happen. I also didn't know how much pathology the angiographer would find and whether he would be able to fix it. So, early in the morning, I called back and asked to be relieved of duty.

Still not knowing when my angiogram would be done, I went to the hospital to tie up a few loose ends—put equipment in my locker, deposit billing slips in our office, and drop by the Cardiac Catheterization Lab to find out the estimated time of my procedure. After that, I planned to go home until it was time to return for my test. By then, Rachel would be back from Arcadia, and we could go together in my car.

Kevin had chosen Dr. Raj Makkar, a highly skilled angiographer, to perform my test. I went to the Cath Lab and heard that Raj's first patient had eaten breakfast.

Patients sometimes misunderstand, forget, or just don't realize the importance of not taking anything by mouth prior to a procedure with anesthesia. Normally when we eat or drink, a piece of soft tissue called the *epiglottis* goes over the *larynx* (voice box), making sure the swallowed material ends up in our stomachs, not our lungs. This mechanism gets disrupted under heavy sedation, and especially by anesthesia. So, if there's anything in the stomach and it gets regurgitated, it can end up in the lungs.

Food particles in the lungs can block an airway, allowing harmful bacteria to grow and multiply in an enclosed space. In addition, stomach acid and digestive enzymes present in the regurgitated food can destroy lung tissue through the same chemical processes they use to break down cells of chicken, broccoli, and everything else we eat. In effect, they can digest a part of the lung. All this can lead to a severe form of pneumonia (called *aspiration pneumonia*), days in an ICU, and even death. Except in an emergency situation such as massive bleeding, in which waiting is even more dangerous than going ahead, procedures with anesthesia are delayed until the stomach has time to empty.

Some patients claim nobody told them not to eat before anesthesia. More likely, they weren't listening carefully, since it's a routine part of pre-op instructions, both oral and written. At any rate, whenever someone eats just prior to a scheduled operation, it means we've had a *Cool Hand Luke*–level of "failure to communicate."

Lots of patients plead, "It was just a tiny sandwich," or an energy bar, or whatever other meal they considered small enough to overlook. But a few chunks of food in the lungs can lead to disaster. Safety trumps convenience.

Everyone involved pays a price for this kind of communication failure. The patient has to come back another day; if staff had started setting up for the procedure prior to cancellation, the hospital ends up throwing away disposable sterile supplies (gauzes, syringes, plastic tubing) and has to re-sterilize instruments; the room may stay empty for hours in the middle of the workday.

Most people don't throw up during or after surgery and anesthesia. Therefore, the majority of patients with a full stomach would probably not aspirate. But the fact that people can often get away with risky behavior is a weak argument. It's like a drunk driver reasoning, "I've driven sloshed before and haven't killed anyone yet."

Because of the breakfast, Raj's first case that day had to be cancelled, opening up a slot of several hours in the schedule, just as I strolled into the Cardiac Cath Lab. Angiography doesn't usually require an anesthesiologist. However other procedures in the Cath Lab, such as the treatment of some arrhythmias, call for heavy sedation with periods of complete anesthesia. I'd done numerous cases in the Cath Lab and knew most of the people who worked there.

After exchanging hellos, I said to the charge nurse, "I am having a cardiac cath myself today."

"Yes, wow! I was surprised to see your name on the add-on list."

"What time do you think my procedure will start?"

"Sometime late in the afternoon, after Dr. Makkar's previously scheduled cases are completed. We don't know for sure when . . . or if you're NPO (*nil per os*, Latin medical jargon for "nothing by mouth"), we can do it right now?"

Not knowing the time of my procedure and wanting to avoid a potential delay, I had taken the precaution of not eating that morning.

Waiting around until an uncertain hour in the late afternoon didn't sound very appealing. I called Rachel to tell her about the new schedule. Already on the freeway on her way to Arcadia, she turned around and headed for the hospital. The change in timing felt abrupt and a bit rushed, but also welcome because it removed an uncertainty in my schedule and moved me closer to the resolution of my problem.

From the lab, I went to the sixth-floor patient check-in area. A clerk asked me questions about my address and insurance, also about wearing seatbelts, receiving flu shots and other trivia that have become part of the admission process. Then she asked, "Would you like an escort to take you to the Cath Lab?"

"Thanks, but no. I know the way."

I used my security badge to open the double doors to the lab and presented myself, along with my paperwork, to the charge nurse who, minutes earlier, had moved my procedure into the gap in the schedule. On numerous other occasions, I had stood at the same desk looking for information on my patients. This time in an unwelcome role reversal, I was directed to get on a gurney. Behind a curtain, I removed my surgical scrubs and put on a patient gown, physically and symbolically transforming my identity. I placed my clothes and doctor's ID badge in a plastic bag labeled with my name and the inscription, PERSONAL BELONGINGS.

As a doctor, I felt at home in the hospital. However, lying on a gurney, as a patient, I felt awkward, out of place, uncomfortable, naked, vulnerable, and a little embarrassed. There was no logical reason to feel embarrassed, but being sick carries a stigma, a feeling that you've done something wrong to get yourself in that situation, no matter how innocent you might be.

In the past, people might have been deemed inadequately pious, meriting punishment for sins. Susan Sontag pointed out in her book *Illness as Metaphor* that tuberculosis was once deemed a disease of excessive sexual passion, with the "tubercular . . . 'consumed' by ardor . . . leading to the dissolution of the body." Sontag also noted that cancer has been blamed on repressed feelings. The prominent psychoanalyst Wilhelm Reich attributed cancer to "emotional resignation," and used Sigmund Freud's oral cancer to demonstrate what repressed sexual feelings can do to a passionate but unhappily married man. Today, we would more likely blame Freud's smoking.

People often go to great lengths to hide their illnesses, to avoid the stigma of weakness. FDR and JFK did that successfully throughout their presidencies. Recently Secretary of Defense Lloyd Austin initially kept his hospitalization for prostate cancer secret from President Biden, the Deputy Secretary of Defense (who temporarily took over his responsibilities), and the public. Ordinary folks may also want to hide an illness to escape loss of esteem and power in their relationships.

When submitting to be a patient, people lose control over their autonomy, allowing others to make decisions for them. They even sign a written permit agreeing to the terms of surrender. With a nurse standing over them, waiting for their signature, virtually no patient reads the multipage text of semi-comprehensible legalese that allows doctors, nurses, and technicians to do whatever. Every patient suffers a loss of power. As a physician, perhaps I felt this even more intensely, going from the highest to the lowest rung in the autonomy hierarchy of the medical setting.

I scanned the permit and quickly wrote my name, reasoning that, "I know what's in these forms," even though I really didn't. I signed, just like everybody else.

A nurse started my IV. Raj asked questions about my medical history and explained what he would do. Several doctors, nurses, and technicians, surprised to hear about my new role, came by to wish me luck and to remark jokingly how confused and tired I must be to lie down on a patient gurney. Their well-intentioned banter helped relieve some of the tension I'd been feeling, letting me focus on our interactions instead of my upcoming test. I had been on the other side of such exchanges many times, whenever I had seen a doctor or nurse friend on a gurney. I welcomed the warm tone and kind intent of this support from my colleagues.

One other thing differentiated my interactions with the staff from that of most patients. The nurses and technicians all addressed me as *Dr.* Kadar. Had I not been a physician, they would almost surely have called me by my first name, the usual custom at Cedars and other hospitals.

By contrast, unless I know them well or they ask me to use their first name, I usually call my patients *Mr., Ms., Mrs.* or *Dr.* We're products of our upbringing, which includes our education. At my medical school at Yale University, the faculty emphasized treating patients with as much dignity as possible. One professor, an impeccably dressed New England gentleman who always wore a bright-colored bow tie in the hospital, memorably said, "Only children, pets, and patients are addressed by their first names on a first encounter. Don't your patients deserve as much respect as any random stranger you meet?" He added that many middle-aged and elderly patients feel uncomfortable being called by their first names by younger hospital personnel. A medical encounter strips people of their clothes and private space. It can strip away our sense of self, as my diagnosis had done, and our sense of agency. It doesn't have to strip away common courtesy and dignity.

The professor who uttered the memorable admonition may have been more accurate for his place and time; we tend to be more informal in California today. Nevertheless, I still think it's important to extend maximal courtesy and respect to my patients. That generally leaves me as the only person in an operating room addressing the patient by his or her last name. I think at least some of them feel more comfortable and respected by that, an outcome worth the effort.

I was wheeled from the prep area into a procedure suite. Raj instructed the monitoring nurse to inject a sedative through my IV. From that moment on, my experience of the angiography and the time it took to complete it disappeared into the fog of sedation. The next thing I remember is Raj telling me in the recovery room that he was going to get a cardiac surgeon to talk to me.

"Did you do an angioplasty? How many vessels?" I asked.

"No. No angioplasty."

"Why not?"

"I'm going to get one of the surgeons to talk to you."

I knew what was coming, even in my post-sedation haze. If a doctor who makes his living doing angioplasties tells you he wants a surgeon to talk to you, it can only mean bad news. Raj's decision not to perform angioplasty was proof positive that he didn't think it would work. Although my doctors still talked about a decision-making process including me, my cardiologist, angiographer, and surgeon, I already knew the final verdict would be that my condition called for open-heart surgery.

Sure enough, that's what Dr. Alfredo Trento, the cardiac surgeon, told me. He said I had significant blockages in three of my coronary arteries and needed to have a three-vessel bypass.

Coronary artery bypass grafting (CABG—pronounced "cabbage") begins with a six-inch incision into the chest, followed by cutting through the breastbone and the sack around the heart (the *pericardium*), and into coronary arteries. All those tissues must heal before the patient can feel well again, a process that takes over three months.

By contrast, angioplasty doesn't require an incision, only a needle stuck through the skin, which heals within hours. The angiographer punctures a large artery (usually one on the right or left side of the groin), guides a long, thin plastic tube (called a *catheter*) from there into the heart, finds a narrowed area in a coronary artery using video X-ray, dilates a balloon that widens the constriction, and places a stent (a plastic or metal scaffold) to keep the vessel open. This less traumatic procedure leads to a much faster, easier recuperation than open-heart surgery. Whenever it can provide an equally good result, angioplasty is the obvious choice.

To understand the situation, we have to look at blood vessel anatomy. The right coronary artery provides oxygenated blood to the cells of the right side of the heart. The left main coronary artery supplies the left side through two principal tributaries. The larger of these, the left anterior descending, distributes blood to the front and bottom of the left side. The other, called the circumflex, supplies the top and rear portions of the left chambers.

Angiographers take video images of these vessels and their tributaries to reveal one of three possible situations: minimal or no occlusions, meaning the patient's symptoms are not due to atherosclerosis; one or more areas of narrowing that can be treated with balloon and stent to restore adequate flow; or occlusions that cannot be dilated by angioplasty. In that latter case, a surgeon enters the picture and CABG becomes the safest treatment.

Kevin described the details of my pathology. The angiograms showed a 70 percent occlusion in the circumflex artery, an 80 percent occlusion in the first portion of the left anterior descending artery, and a 99 percent blockage in the right coronary artery. Any coronary artery narrowing greater than 50 percent poses an increased risk of a heart attack. Three of the largest arteries supplying both sides of my heart had occlusions that handily exceeded that threshold. The left anterior descending artery supplies oxygenated blood to the largest amount of heart tissue. Its narrowing posed the greatest risk. Its' blockage causes sudden death from fatal heart attacks so often that it's referred to as the "widow maker." Certain that Rachel would cringe to hear the term "widow maker," I decided not to mention it to her.

The discussions with Kevin and Alfredo each lasted only a few minutes, long enough to clarify the situation and seal the verdict. I had been included in the discussion, but my illness limited my options. The pattern of my pathology wiped out the prospect of a successful angioplasty in multiple ways. First, three-vessel occlusions require three different dilations that must each stay open, nearly tripling the chance of ending up with an obstructed artery. Second, the opening in the 99 percent occluded right coronary artery was smaller than the diameter of the balloon-tipped catheter, even in its uninflated state. In order to pass the catheter into that segment, the channel would first have to be widened by destroying a portion of the plaque with bursts of laser beams. That can damage the vessel wall and even perforate it, increasing the procedure's risk since my surgery. (Further advances in technology since my surgery now make it easier to stent a 99 percent occluded coronary artery.) Finally, the "widow maker" narrowing in the left anterior descending (LAD) coronary artery responds poorly to angioplasty, frequently closing off afterward and leading to a massive heart attack. If the narrowing had been farther down, somewhere in the midcourse of my LAD, the lesion could have been ballooned. But dilating this artery at its root is technically difficult and produces a high risk of the pathology living up to its scary nickname.

As I wrote earlier, I realized what was coming as soon as Raj said, "No angioplasty." I didn't know the details then, but big, bad surgery looked inevitable. After the first huge "oh crap" moment, I felt resigned to what needed to be done. I trusted my doctors. Having worked at the same hospital, I had the advantage of knowing for certain that they were all very capable. These were the doctors I would want to take care of me if I was sick . . . and oh yes, damn it, I was sick. For the first time in my life, I had a disease that could kill me. Not a great situation, but one that could have a happy outcome. *I'm going to be okay.*

The best advice I can give to anybody contemplating open-heart surgery, or any other major treatment, is to find a hospital and doctors you can trust. The outcome can never be guaranteed, but being in good hands in a good place tilts the odds in the patient's favor . . . as much as possible.

My first angina wake-up whisper had arrived a mere nine days earlier. Fully convinced that I had no heart disease, I could have easily ignored mild chest burning after strenuous exercise, blaming it on heartburn. Even with my medical background, I did nothing about it until the third episode. But that incident was also mild enough to be ignored, except for my inner doctor directing me to err on the side of caution. Did that save my life? Would I have sought help in time if I hadn't been so familiar with the symptoms of coronary artery disease? That's hard to know, since the time sequence from first symptom to a fatal event can vary so much. The two subsequent recurrences of chest pain with normal daily activities were more disturbing. These episodes put me in the lucky half of those with serious heart issues who receive a forewarning and an opportunity to seek treatment.

I say that with a lot of hesitation. The tendency to call somebody with a horrible illness "lucky" has always struck me as bizarre.

When I was a surgery intern at University of California, San Diego, a 30-something woman arrived in the emergency room with a large kitchen knife sticking out of her abdomen, just below her belly button. One-third of the broad nine-inch blade protruded from her body and was topped by a six-inch wooden handle, standing straight up like a flagpole. With the rest of the blade hidden from our view, there was no way to know what damage pulling the knife out might cause. If the blade had nicked a blood vessel on the way in, it might be acting as a plug keeping massive amounts of blood from pouring out. If it had cut into a section of bowel, it could be keeping feces from seeping into the abdomen. The safest course was to leave the knife in place until her belly was opened, and remove it under direct visualization.

Prepping the abdomen for sterility presented an unusual problem. The nurse poured a golden-brown iodine solution over the knife handle, letting the liquid slide down over the blade and onto the patient's abdomen. The lead surgeon made the skin incision and carefully worked his way down the course of the blade, noting that it had penetrated the small intestine in several places and barely missed her *aorta*, the largest artery.

One of the residents remarked. "Boy, she sure is lucky. A quarter of an inch to the left, that knife would have cut her aorta."

If that had happened, she would have bled to death before reaching the hospital. This woman didn't die on the spot; instead, she just had a five-inch-wide incision in her abdomen and intestinal contents that had spilled throughout her belly. The cut and the spillage led to inflammation called *peritonitis* and several weeks of pain, fever, and disability while she recovered from surgery. In addition, she doubtlessly suffered mental anguish from the memory of attempted murder by her "boyfriend." I doubt that many of us envy her "luck."

Since then, I've participated in numerous operations on patients with major trauma from auto crashes, industrial accidents, and bullet wounds. Invariably, somebody remarks how "lucky" the patient is. When it's a gun injury, it's usually because if the bullet had traversed one inch over, it would have hit a big blood vessel and the victim would be dead already. What nonsense! If those patients had really been lucky, they wouldn't have been shot.

Getting angina is certainly better than getting shot or suffering a massive heart attack, but good fortune is relative. My situation could surely have been worse. However, I had taken a "bullet" and dealing with it called for a major operation, pain, at least temporary disability, and a risk of complications. That didn't sound like wonderful luck to me.

Nevertheless, in some respects I was lucky: my warnings didn't kill me. A first episode of angina in an otherwise healthy individual, particularly if the pain is mild, stands the risk of being ignored or rationalized away. It certainly was by me, even though I would never ignore a presentation like mine from one of my patients. Psychologists call this phenomenon the "incredulity response." It happens whenever people see something wrong, even a danger like a building on fire or a gunman on the loose, but just cannot accept that what they are seeing is real.

For example, a fire broke out in the London subway system at King's Cross station in 1987. Trains continued to arrive and commuters in a hurry continued to board them, even as others frantically escaped the smoke and flames. Thirty-one people died.

I can be faulted for my denial since, as a doctor, I should have known better. However, the symptoms of heart attack are familiar enough to the general public that even people who don't work in medicine should know better.

Mr. A, a 50-year-old man, for example, developed severe chest pain while driving home from a ski trip. The pain radiated to his jaw and left arm, classic symptoms of cardiac ischemia. When he also started having profuse sweating and dizziness, his wife took over the wheel and drove to an emergency room. His electrocardiogram showed a pattern of depressions indicative of a large heart attack. Nevertheless, he insisted that he was fit, couldn't possibly be having a heart attack, and refused to put on a hospital gown in preparation for going to the cardiac catheterization suite.

The majority of people who die from a heart attack do so without getting medical care. Had it not been for his wife, Mr. A might very well have joined their ranks. In this case, however, he relented to cardiac catheterization and received a successful angioplasty while still wearing his street clothes.

With the aid of his wife and insistent medical personnel, Mr. A managed to receive prompt treatment despite his denial. But many others don't. Their refusal to acknowledge reality leads to delays in intervention that result in preventable deaths. So, the take-home message is this—don't ignore or rationalize away chest pain. If it's severe and persistent pain and especially if it comes on with exercise and ceases promptly with rest, don't let incredulity cost you your life.

Like so many at the King's Cross station, I found it difficult to acknowledge the unexpected, to accept bad news I didn't want to believe. Fortunately, I had enough time and took enough precaution to get off the wrong track and take the first step to getting better: getting a diagnosis.

My story so far has centered on denial. This phenomenon delays medical treatment often enough to give rise to the cliche that "Denial is not just a river in Egypt."

People with major psychiatric problems notoriously refuse to acknowledge their afflictions. Such denial can result in self-destructive decisions, out-of-control addictions, and even suicide.

Denial malignantly postpones cancer treatment: *This lump is not so hard. It's not so big. Just a bruise. It'll go away.* Even when the diagnosis is certain, hesitation can put off therapy long enough to reduce the prospect of a cure. Steve Jobs, the genius who conceived and helped deliver so many amazing Apple innovations, was diagnosed with early-stage cancer, apparently still confined in his pancreas. He delayed potentially curative surgery for nine months. Jobs eventually had a cancer resection operation and a subsequent liver transplant, but only after his tumor had spread. Ultimately it killed him at the age of 56. According to his biographer, Walter Isaacson, Jobs "felt that if you ignore something, if you don't want something to exist, you can have magical thinking." Denial thrives on such fantasy.

One version of "magical thinking" inspires blind faith in the alleged miraculous power of traditional healing practices. These come in a variety of shapes and from all corners of the world—high in the Andes or Himalayas, deep in the rainforests of Central America or Africa, from Native American healers, and from purveyors of "new age technology" developed in Europe or the USA.

Denial can culminate in sudden death, even for someone as focused on promoting good heath as Jim Fixx (although in his case, we don't know for sure whether he had any prior symptoms). It can produce profound regret and necessitate more drastic and less-effective surgery, even for someone as brilliant as Steve Jobs. Or you can be lucky enough to arrive at acceptance in time to receive treatment that has the best chance to produce a favorable outcome.

Chapter 3

Embracing Your New Reality:
The Power of Acceptance

To the dumb question "Why me?" the cosmos
barely bothers to return the reply: Why not.

—Christopher Hitchens, *Mortality*

Acceptance and initiating treatment can reduce stress and anxiety as the situation is better understood, even with remaining uncertainties. Knowing the enemy is the first step to confronting it. Plans can be drawn, and treatment can begin.

Some people embrace the new clarity. Literary critic Anatole Broyard wrote that he "felt something like relief, even elation, when the doctor told me that I had cancer of the prostate." He embraced the drama of the crisis. His mindset was altered to such a degree that he felt *Intoxicated by My Illness,* the title he chose for his book. It should be noted that Broyard was writing about his reaction upon receiving the diagnosis. At the time, he didn't believe the cancer was going to kill him. Fourteen months later it did.

The awareness that a dreaded diagnosis has been confirmed can also increase worry. After all, deadly diseases can be just that—deadly. But not always. Treatments can cure the disease or at least extend life by many years. People hope . . . and pray.

Regarding public speaking, television newscaster Walter Cronkite opined that, "It's natural to have butterflies. The secret is to get them to fly in formation." Controlling the fear and anxiety generated by a medical crisis calls for a similar trick.

It's not a secret that a positive attitude helps you in life. Mayo Clinic reports that the health benefits of a positive attitude may include:

- Increased life span
- Lower rates of depression
- Lower levels of distress and pain
- Greater resistance to illnesses
- Better psychological and physical well-being
- Better cardiovascular health and reduced risk of death from cardiovascular disease and stroke
- Reduced risk of death from cancer
- Reduced risk of death from respiratory conditions
- Reduced risk of death from infections
- Better coping skills during hardships and times of stress[1]

In a study of over 70,000 women, Harvard's T.H. Chan School of Public Health found that women with optimistic attitudes had a 30 percent lower risk of dying from a number of diseases than women with significantly less optimistic attitudes.[2]

Yet Steve Jobs' optimistic "magical thinking" clearly did not help. There's a difference between magical thinking and a positive attitude. Professor Martin Hagger of Curtin University, the author of a study on positive attitudes,[3] said that "what people think about their illness impacts on what they will do about it and, importantly, their recovery, or, at least, how well they manage their illness." Hagger added that "people who view their illness as more serious and symptomatic, and have strong negative emotions about it, were more likely to adopt avoidance or go into denial to cope. Those people are also more likely to experience depression and anxiety, and they are less likely to get better."[4]

At 8:55 a.m. that Wednesday, I was transferred from the Angio Suite to a recovery room. An hour later, a second move landed me in the Coronary Care Unit with the diagnosis of "unstable angina." This implied that even a minor exertion could cause *cardiac ischemia* (decreased blood flow) and a heart attack. Despite that, I had no discomfort resting in bed and thought that my diagnosis sounded much worse than I felt. I suffered from a life-threatening disease and had accepted what needed to be done. However, it seemed odd, puzzling, even mildly amusing, that I could be so sick but not feel sick at all.

I had walked into Dr. Drury's office on Tuesday afternoon for my stress test. Less than a day later, I was told that my operation, a triple-vessel coronary artery bypass graft, was already on the schedule for 7:15 a.m. the following morning. The time from the first diagnostic test to the start of open-heart surgery was a mere day and a half. Events were moving so fast I hardly had enough time to worry.

Illness and recovery proceeds at its own pace. That's something nearly all of us have to face sometime, along with the accompanying uncertainty.

Perhaps I should have been more anxious, but my default mode tends to be optimism.

The afternoon before my surgery, I didn't feel completely calm, but I was more apprehensive than fearful. A large incision in the chest produces significant, sometimes excruciating pain. The shock to the body from a major operation causes weakness. Although the odds of surviving the surgery were strongly in my favor, the prospect of some level of disability afterward posed a greater risk. In particular, I wondered, *Will I be able to continue my career?*

Some open-heart surgery patients suffer brain damage, including memory loss and decreased thinking ability, the capacity to process information and solve problems. Cognitive deficit following a cardiac bypass, called *postperfusion syndrome* in professional journals and "pump head" in medical locker-room jargon, continues to be the subject of evolving debate and research. Opinions about its cause and incidence and whether it is transient or permanent remain controversial.

What if the operation changes me? An anesthesiologist needs to be able to think quickly and respond promptly to a variety of changing conditions. In the middle of an operation, if a patient's blood pressure goes too high or too low, if he or she develops a cardiac arrhythmia, has rapid blood loss, a decrease in oxygenation or suffers any one of numerous other potential setbacks, prompt reaction saves the day. Delay can lead to catastrophe. Anesthesiologists cannot function with either a memory deficit or slowed ability to evaluate and respond to their patient's condition, which can change rapidly during the course of an operation.

I also didn't want to be less intelligent in other realms of my life. Coping with daily challenges is difficult enough with my brain intact. How well would I function if a portion of it went out of commission? How I lived my life, interacted with others, learned new information and skills, and my self-image were all in jeopardy. Dwelling on that was not going to help. Adopting an attitude of facing the challenge head-on and pursuing the best possible outcome would make the best possible outcome more likely. That's the mindset I determined to embrace and slipped into.

I dismissed the idea of dying. I was aware, of course, that severe triple-vessel disease is life-threatening, that I had a coronary artery occlusion deadly enough to be called the "widow maker." But I also knew that the people who suddenly drop dead are rarely asymptomatic patients under continuous electrocardiographic monitoring in a CCU. I tried to focus on the knowledge that I was under the care of a well-trained team who, like me, wanted the best possible outcome.

The fact that I had no pain, no distress at all, also reassured me. I figured that if I rested until surgery and didn't do anything strenuous, my heart would continue to receive enough nourishment and I would remain safe.

Of course, even without exertion, ischemic heart disease can take a sudden turn for the worse. A plaque in a coronary artery can break off, precipitate clotting, and block the artery completely, causing a heart attack. A bad enough heart attack could lead to ventricular fibrillation, a fatal arrhythmia. But I was in the CCU, where cardiopulmonary resuscitation (CPR) would be started promptly. Mulling over the odds, I felt it was most unlikely that anything bad would happen to me before surgery, and even if something did, I was in the best possible place to have it treated.

Did my knowledge of this disease process reduce my apprehension? It could just as easily have increased it. I knew very well that my pathology had the power to trigger sudden death. Perhaps thinking about it in the abstract made it easier for me to cope, by letting me intellectualize the situation and feel a bit more detached from the threat to my life. Or maybe it was just the easiest technique to buttress my denial.

Refusing to acknowledge obvious symptoms before the diagnosis is made leads to delay in seeking lifesaving intervention and is dangerous. However, in patients already hospitalized and awaiting heart surgery, denial can produce positive effects by lowering anxiety and the incidence of depression. Anxiety increases heart rate and raises blood pressure, forcing the heart to work harder. Depression saps energy, the will to live and the motivation to work to promote recovery. An attitude of relative tranquility can actually reduce danger.

Midafternoon in the CCU, I got a phone call from my colleague who made out our schedules. He asked me whom I wanted to do my anesthesia. All of our cardiac anesthesiologists are very capable, and I would have been comfortable with any of them. Given the choice, I picked Dr. Nicola D'Attellis, who is not only highly skilled but also radiates warmth and empathy. Nic was then in his early 50s. Originally from Montreal, he had come to Cedars after serving as the Director of Cardiothoracic Anesthesia at a major hospital in Paris, France.

Most anesthesiologists, including me, wear scrubs whenever they're in the hospital. Nic arrived in my room for the pre-op visit in a navy-blue sports coat that complements his dark hair. Standing to the right of my bed, facing Rachel and me, he asked a series of questions that make up an anesthetic history. "What operations have you had in the past? What type of anesthesia with each? Any anesthetic problems? Allergies, medications, smoking and alcohol use, any other medical diagnoses or symptoms?" Then he explained the anesthetic procedure he planned to use and gave us a chance to ask him questions.

"Will the perfusionist use high flow or low flow?" I asked.

"He'll use the right amount of flow," Nic replied with a smile and a sympathetic nod.

I had asked a question that doesn't occur to many patients, just ones who read medical journals. Most patients worry in broad terms about the unknown dangers they will face during a major operation. Doctor patients aren't immune from fearing the unknown, but we can also focus our apprehension on specific known complications. A doctor doesn't forget everything he or she knows when they check in as a patient. We don't stop being doctors.

I knew that the ideal flow rate from the heart-lung machine used during bypass surgery has been a subject of research, debate, and controversy. The surgeon decides the rate, and the perfusionist controls the dials that regulate it. Some scientists have speculated that differences in flow rates may account for variation in the incidence of post-operative brain problems.

Nic understood my concern. He advised me to relax and let others do the driving this time. An anesthesiologist's training centers on being on top of the situation, aware of everything important to the patient's safety during surgery. Nic was asking me to stop being my usual self. He was asking me to be the patient, not the doctor. I knew he was right; I had to trust my doctors. I also knew that I had good reason to trust them. They were all excellent in their fields and my operation would take place in an outstanding hospital.

I didn't ask any other technical questions. After a few reassuring words, Nic mentioned that the best way to get well rapidly and avoid complications was to be active right after surgery.

"Get out of bed and walk as much as you can."

He was preaching to the choir. Before I went to medical school, I believed that doctors routinely exaggerated the amount of time it takes to recover from an injury. Guys on my UCLA Gymnastics teams got back in the gym in half the time they were told it would take to heal. Early in my medical education, I learned that my gymnast sample was not representative of all patients. Highly motivated college athletes tend to recover faster than average, due to their youth, fitness, and eagerness to return to competition.

I'm also aware of the dangers and limitations of thinking that way. No matter how ideal your mindset and fitness, some injuries and illnesses are fatal. Magical thinking that the patient determines the outcome can add an extra burden of guilt on someone who cannot recover from a catastrophic disease such as metastatic cancer.

Nevertheless, in my mind I remained a young gymnast who could bounce back from any injury in record time. When Nic emphasized the importance of early ambulation in promoting recovery, I was primed and ready, determined to walk better and faster after a CABG than just about anybody who had ever had one.

Shortly before 7:00 a.m. the next day, an orderly arrived in my room. I knew him well from the many times he'd helped transport my patients, bringing them to a pre-op area and taking them to a recovery room or an ICU.

"Ready, Doc? . . . Or would you like a few more minutes with your family?"

"I'm ready, David. Let's roll."

Hospital rules permit one family member to stay in the pre-operative area with the patient. Rachel sat by my right side. In an echo of the pre-angio scenario, a parade of anesthesiologists, surgeons, nurses, and techs visited me briefly with some variation of the by-now-familiar "Aren't you on the wrong side of the bed, Doctor?" and "Good luck!"

I appreciated the camaraderie. I was in good hands. The odds were in my favor. *This is just something I have to get through,* I thought. *No other choice.*

Focusing on the people around me helped.

Whenever we were left alone, Rachel and I continued our attempts to reassure each other. We held hands and punctuated that connection with an occasional squeeze, including our secret pattern of squeezes that mean "I love you."

Nic arrived with a cardiac anesthesiology fellow and a resident. Cedars-Sinai is a teaching hospital. As the attending physician, Nic functioned as both a clinician and a teacher, performing some of the procedures personally and supervising the fellow and resident. Though still completing their formal education, residents and fellows are knowledgeable and capable enough to make the attending's job easier.

Soon afterward, Alfredo Trento, my surgeon, looking dapper as usual in a perfectly fitted stylish gray suit, came by to say hello. Italian by birth, Alfredo complements his obvious surgical skills with Old World charm and abundant panache. After he left, Rachel remarked, "That doctor could be a model for a fashion magazine."

A few minutes later, with all personnel ready to go, Nic returned to tell me it was time for the main event. Rachel and I exchanged a final hug and kiss. Then she watched as the nurses and anesthesiologists started to roll my gurney toward the operating room. Looking backward over my shoulder, I could see Rachel fighting back tears.

My new entourage escorted me down the back corridor. My predominant emotion was not fear but amazement—mixed with outrage. My inner voice kept screaming: *This should not be happening to me!* As we entered the OR, the screams faded with the onset of the soothing effects of sedation.

As noted, resilience and a positive attitude are crucial to reaching a good outcome to a medical crisis. Those who expect to do poorly tend to fulfill their own expectations. Patients who don't push themselves to do well often don't. Recovery is a team effort requiring everyone to play their part. Of course, doctors, nurses, and therapists have to provide appropriate care, but the patient's determination, attitude, and mindset remain crucial factors.

Some surgeons and anesthesiologists will cancel an operation if a patient declares the belief that they will die during the procedure. Expressing a desire not to wake up after surgery rings another loud alarm. I'm not sure if there is any data on this, nor how it could be collected, but there is a feeling that expectation of death increases the risk of it coming to pass. At the very least, a patient who wants to die is unlikely to strive to do what he or she needs to do to help themself recuperate. When pain and exhaustion hit, motivating a person who has given up may pose an insurmountable obstacle. Refusal to make the effort to walk in the post-operative period increases the likelihood of forming blood clots in the legs. Those clots can travel as *emboli* to the lungs and deliver the fatal ending the patient expected.

The puzzle has many parts, but a determined and hopeful attitude is a crucial piece. It's an approach worth cultivating prior to entering an operating room. A supportive loved one in pre-op, someone also dedicated to the patient's recovery, reinforces the necessary positive vibe.

Chapter 4

Turning Points: Surgery and the Miracles of Modern Medicine

> Extreme remedies are very appropriate for extreme disease.
>
> —Hippocrates

Since the events of the operating room took place after I felt the first effects of sedation, I don't recall any of them. Though people often refer to anesthesia as sleep, and patients under anesthesia may look like they're asleep, anesthesia is a very different state. If someone were to cut into the chest of a sleeping person, he or she would immediately wake up screaming in agony and might take a protective swing at their assailant. Anesthesia enables surgeons to cut into muscle, saw bones, and take as much time as needed to remove diseased organs.

Before the introduction of modern anesthesia, surgery was a brutal affair, requiring six strong men to hold down a terrified patient as the knife descended. The range of operations was limited to procedures that needed to be done badly enough that patients were willing to submit to such torture—active bleeding, trauma injuries, amputations, and excising visible tumors. Speed was of the essence to limit the duration of the excruciating assault. You may have seen old Western movies in which a patient guzzles a bottle of whiskey before surgery. Sometimes patients did drink alcohol or were given narcotics to dull sensation, but attempting to eliminate pain entirely with those agents risked causing the person to die from intoxication.

The first public demonstration of effective surgical anesthesia with ether (in 1846, at the Massachusetts General Hospital in Boston) changed the world of medicine. With anesthesia giving them more time and patients who held still instead of writhing in agony, surgeons were able to develop operations to treat a far wider range of maladies.

Anesthetics cause unconsciousness. Throughout a surgery, anesthesiologists have the responsibility to keep patients alive and pain-free. That requires constant attention to heart rate and rhythm, blood pressure, oxygenation, temperature, blood loss, fluid infusion, urine output, and other factors that vary with procedures. The head of an anesthesiologist moves like the periscope of a submarine, always scanning the field for anything that requires intervention. The sooner a problem is detected, the easier it is to resolve.

Thursday, November 4

Seconds before we moved out of pre-op, the anesthesiology fellow injected midazolam into my IV. Better known by its brand name of Versed, this drug belongs to a class of sedatives called benzodiazepines. Diazepam, brand name Valium, is another well-known and commonly used member of this class. I refer to Versed as Vitamin V2, since

I give it to my patients every day. I used to call Valium, the most commonly used premedication before the introduction of Versed in the late 1970s, Vitamin V (I've updated that to V1). Versed possesses two advantages over its older cousin: a shorter duration of action and less pain at the injection site. In addition to sedation, benzodiazepines can produce amnesia. Most people don't remember anything after floating into "midazoland," a mythical calm sanctuary that precedes the storm of surgery. Many ask when we are going to begin surgery as they emerge from anesthesia after multi-hour procedures.

As patients, we don't go through surgery alone. The medical team is with us and, if we're lucky, a loved one. One influential research project found, "Surgical patients with a strong network of friends & family reported better scores for anxiety, depression, inner peace, relaxation, pain intensity and pain unpleasantness for every day of the five post-surgical follow-up days. They needed fewer painkillers and were less likely than other patients to stay in the hospital longer than 7 days."[1]

For me, the linchpin of that support was Rachel. The next section of this chapter is Rachel's firsthand account of her experiences on the day of my operation.

After you disappeared around the corner on the way to the operating room, Walter, one of the cardiac surgery nurses, guided me to the sixth-floor waiting lounge. I took a seat next to a tall, dark-green, leafy plant near a window.

A dozen or so others in the lounge appeared lost in private thoughts, their faces obscured behind magazines or cell phones. An equal number engaged in hushed conversations, interrupted by long pauses, staring at the ground, and an occasional sigh. Several men and women were bleary-eyed. Some appeared to be struggling to keep their eyes open, closing them for a few seconds at a time. A few yawned; others stifled yawns. One woman was lying on a couch, eyes closed, a beige blanket covering her. One man was nervously tapping his feet. Whenever someone came through the door from the surgical corridor, everyone's eyes anxiously darted in that direction. They all appeared to be on tenterhooks, eagerly awaiting news about their loved ones.

I must have looked that way. All my mind craved at that moment was for time to speed up and for you to emerge safely from surgery. To distract myself, I reached for one of the magazines strewn atop a nearby end table and absentmindedly scanned three-month-old news of celebrities' shenanigans.

At one point, a hospital volunteer in her 70s named Helen approached me and asked if Dr. Kadar was my husband. After hearing my reply, Helen said, "He took care of me seven years ago when I had arm surgery. He was gentle and caring. I liked the way he treated me. He's a very good doctor and a very good man."

I thanked Helen for her kind words. Throughout the morning, I continued to be preoccupied with worry. I feared something bad would happen, that you might even die. You'd told me the odds were on our side and that after recuperating, you would be your previous self. That didn't keep me from thinking about a bad outcome. Helen's comment unleashed a torrent of thoughts.

I've got to do all I can to keep my husband alive. I love him and need him. And now he needs me. He is a good man. I'm not going to let go of him. I need to make him healthy. I'm not gonna let go.

I couldn't help but recall an old Chinese prejudice. A woman whose husband died shortly after their wedding used to be condemned as a "super scissor," a toxic instrument responsible for cutting her husband's life short. Such women were shunned. They could never marry again. Some were even killed—drowned in a river or stoned to death.

Logically, I could dismiss such a stupid, archaic, misogynistic superstition. But I had heard about it ever since I was a little girl and knew that all my Chinese friends would recall it as well. The thought of being labeled a super scissor, even of conjuring up the idea, tormented me. It reinforced my determination for the notion that reverberated over and over in my mind that day, *I'm not going to let go of him. I'm NOT gonna let go.*

During the operation, Walter kept me apprised of progress, periodically coming to the waiting room to reassure me that everything was proceeding according to plan. Around 9:00 a.m., he told me the prep was over and a short time later that the incision had been made. At noon, Walter returned with the news that you were off bypass and surgery would soon be completed. He told me the doctors had found "nothing unexpected." He also gave me an information booklet on coronary artery bypass surgery.

Walter advised me to eat a good lunch, available in the coffee shop or the cafeteria. But I worried that I might be away when Dr. Trento came out to talk to me. I bought a bag of potato chips from a nearby vending machine instead. I didn't have much of an appetite and soon realized I was too nervous to eat. After slowly munching on five or six chips, I threw the rest of the bag in the trash.

An hour later, Walter returned to tell me the operation was over. He led me to Dr. Trento's office for a more detailed update.

I waited there anxiously for half an hour. When Trento finally appeared, he bounded in, still wearing scrubs under a long white coat. He ebulliently told me that everything had gone well.

I felt relieved, but I wanted to know what bad developments could still happen.

"He might need a blood transfusion," Trento said.

A transfusion didn't sound too bad. It was far from my worst fears earlier in the day.

After Trento's reassuring words, Walter escorted me to the CSICU (Cardiac Surgery Intensive Care Unit). The instant I saw you there, I was shocked. Tears gushed from my eyes. You were unconscious and unmoving, ghostly pale, with an intimidating jumble of tubes and wires going in and out of you. There was blood in a container below the bed. The overhead monitor beeped with every beat of your heart, and the ventilator hissed with each breath. You looked so helpless and fragile. The whole scene was scary.

Your ICU room measured about 15 feet by 15 feet, with a floor-to-ceiling clear plastic wall on the side leading to the counters of the nursing station. Half that wall functioned as a sliding glass door, providing a tall and wide opening for hospital beds and equipment. Standing outside your room, nurses and doctors had an aquarium view of all the equipment and activity inside. The head of your bed was positioned at the far wall, with monitors, IV poles, the ventilator, and other medical equipment above and on both sides. The scene exuded sterile functionality and high-tech efficiency. At the back of the room on your right side, there was a small bathroom with a sink, a toilet, and just enough space between them to turn around.

Over the next couple of hours, you opened your eyes, moved your arms and legs, and started breathing on your own. Finally, Dr. D'Attellis removed the breathing tube and asked you, "Andy, do you know me? Do you know who I am?"

You stared at him with a blank expression, eyes wide open. Your pupils were huge, big black circles with barely any blue around them. Your mouth was open, but you didn't say anything, as if you didn't understand the question. I was worried. I wondered why you just glared silently, why you didn't seem to recognize Nic.

He pointed to your nurse. "Do you know who he is?"

You turned slightly but still said nothing. Nic next pointed to me. "Andy, do you know who she is?"

You slowly moved your head to look at me and then, with a weak, barely audible, raspy voice, said, "My wife."

Tears burst from my eyes. It sounds crazy but that was an important moment for me. I thought, *No matter what, he knows me. I must be his true love.*

Nic turned to me and said, "He'll be all right."

Every few minutes throughout the afternoon, you groaned and grimaced in pain. Your erratic, disoriented moaning made me cry. You asked to go to the bathroom many times. The nurse kept explaining that a catheter was emptying your bladder and you could pee without wetting yourself. In a croaky voice, you told me, "Rachel, I want to go home." The farthest we got on that project was dangling your legs by the side of the bed.

Your nurse convinced me to go home and get some rest by saying I would be better able to help you the next day if I did. I left at 11:00 p.m. The drive home felt lonely and our empty home even more so. Despite feeling exhausted, I tossed and turned in bed. My mind was racing with worry. It took me a long time to fall asleep.

Surgeons know that spouses long to hear good news after waiting apprehensively for an operation to conclude. Whenever procedures go well, which they nearly always do, surgeons reassure patients' loved ones by telling them how pleased they are with the results. Alfredo Trento is particularly good at performing this task, naturally radiating confidence and buoyant optimism. (When an operation doesn't go so well, his demeanor is obviously more somber.)

Although Alfredo told Rachel that I might need a transfusion, I managed to avoid it. Transfusions are quite common during and after heart operations. In addition to surgical bleeding, I lost blood in the heart-lung machine. The pump's tubing needs to be primed—filled with nearly three pints of a clear, balanced-salt solution—diluting the blood passing through it. The perfusionist returns as much of the blood as possible at the end of bypass, but the volume retained in the machine results in the loss of at least one pint. My hematocrit (blood count) slipped down from a normal 43 before surgery to 28, a loss of more than one-third of my red blood cells.

The blood loss would have been even greater but for the cell saver. Blood suctioned off the surgical field circulates through this machine, to be processed and made safe for return to the patient. I received one and a half pints of my own blood back that way.

Of course, a transfusion is far from the worst thing that can occur after open-heart surgery. More serious setbacks include stroke, a large blood clot to the lung *(pulmonary embolus)*, heart attack, and even death. By naming the most probable adverse event—the possible need for a transfusion—and not talking about the less likely, more terrifying ones, in my opinion, Alfredo gave Rachel the right answer.

Neither doctors nor ethicists have come to a universal consensus about precisely how much to say to patients and their families. The same approach will certainly not work best in all situations, since the amount of detail ideal for one family can be too much or too little for another.

In my specialty, we meet some patients who want an in-depth explanation of the pros and cons of different anesthetic techniques, along with an enumeration of every gory risk. Others prefer the bliss of not knowing any of that. "Just do what's best for me, Doc," they'll say. I conclude my pre-operative explanations by asking patients and their next of kin if they have any questions for me. Then I can go into as much detail as they want.

In the past, doctors often avoided the C-word, telling cancer patients that they suffered from another, less dread-inducing disease. I had an uncle in Hungary who was a doctor. When he was dying of cancer in the 1960s, his doctors kept insisting that he had a different disease. "I lied to my patients for years that they didn't have cancer. Now you're lying to me just the same way," he declared. His doctors still resisted confirming the truth he already knew. Nevertheless, my uncle received the best available treatment for his illness, which then was palliative care to minimize pain and discomfort.

In the United States today, the medical community's consensus holds that approach to be paternalistic and dishonest, depriving patients of information they can use to plan the rest of their lives. Those who disagree argue that informing people they have a fatal illness is cruel, causes fear and despair, and diminishes the happiness of their remaining days. I believe physicians need to listen to what their patients tell them and never say anything untrue, but not overburden people with detailed information they don't want to hear.

In the past, doctors have also been known to exaggerate dangers. Medical students everywhere hear about an old-time surgeon who enumerated to every patient a long list of horrible complications that could occur during their operations. Then he basked in their admiration when none of those catastrophes came to pass. This story seems likely to be an urban legend. Otherwise, one of these characters must have been practicing in just about every hospital in the country.

Every medical procedure, indeed, every action including getting out of bed in the morning or staying in bed all day, carries a risk. The ultimate risk of anything and everything is, of course, death. Some physicians mention that to their patients prior to any operation. I believe bringing up death when it's very unlikely generates unnecessary anxiety. We may know that the ultimate complication of crossing a street is death, but we rarely think or talk about it before stepping off the curb. If death is specifically discussed, patients may fear it out of proportion to the actual risk.

The majority of American physicians today adhere to a policy of describing what is likely to happen, and adding the most common complications when asked. We believe in treating patients like adults, informing them honestly and realistically, letting their feedback guide the extent of detail enumerated.

A photo Rachel took in the ICU showed my *endotracheal* tube (used to keep the airway open and provide breathing assistance from a ventilator) secured firmly in place, with one-inch-wide silk surgical tape neatly circling its base and extending to the area above my lips and beyond, from ear to ear. A BIS monitor strip, used to record brain waves during surgery, still covered my forehead, although no longer serving any purpose. The container with blood in it collected drainage from my chest tubes.

Years ago, a patient in my situation would have remained on the ventilator overnight, maybe even for several days. Current practice encourages fast tracking—taking out the tube (called *extubation*) within the first eight hours after surgery, for patients who can safely tolerate it. Under this protocol, the amount of ventilatory support provided is gradually decreased. As patients breathe more on their own, they eventually reach the point of no longer needing mechanical help. Doctors can then safely remove the tube. Nic, who also worked as an ICU doctor, took mine out in less than three hours—not unusual, but a sign of very good progress.

With the tube no longer between my vocal cords, I could talk again. Nic asked me to identify him and others to gauge my level of alertness right after extubation. Score one for groggy me, drugged up but still able to recognize my wife.

A catheter puts pressure on the bladder outlet, making people feel like they need to pee, even though a properly functioning catheter empties the bladder. Try explaining that to a sleepy, disoriented patient.

Due to all the drugs I received, the last thing I personally remember from the day of surgery was being wheeled into the operating room and drifting into the soothing haze of premedication. All I know about the immediate post-surgical events comes from what Rachel told me and from reviewing my chart. As a result, I can only speculate about what happened during that night. No doubt I slept restlessly, asked to go to the bathroom a few times, and, with a weak, hoarse voice, requested pain medicine.

As stated before, illness is a family affair. Although only my body was on the operating table, Rachel also experienced trauma that day.

Family members begin the day of surgery with hours of anxiety. Away from their loved one, they worry about something going amiss during the operation. Those worries are compounded by additional ones about how the patient will be changed and how the outcome might affect their own lives.

After surgery, seeing a loved one moaning in pain, separated from the patient by the technology of modern medicine, fearful of doing something harmful while maneuvering around all that equipment, takes a toll. Machines in an ICU, and a mélange of tubes and wires, blood from drains and on dressings, look frightening to someone not used to such a sight. The hissing of the ventilator, the rhythmic beeping of the ECG machine, and an occasional harsh alarm all sound ominous. Most alarms are triggered by a harmless and easily fixable disconnection of a piece of monitoring equipment, but they can momentarily terrify a visitor already on edge. Blood loss makes some patients look ghostly white. The sight of a previously vigorous loved one looking so fragile and in such a precarious state can be surprising and scary. Despite reassurance from doctors and nurses that everything is going well, loved ones often fear that the situation is worse than they're told. They worry about what comes next. The idea that the patient may die lurks in the back of their minds.

PART II

INITIAL RECOVERY
(IN THE HOSPITAL)

Chapter 5

Awakening:
The Dawn of Recovery

A journey of a thousand miles begins with
one step.

—credited to both Confucius and Lao Tzu

The first sensation patients recall after a long operation is often confusion replaced quickly by sharp
pain. Sedation from lingering anesthesia and pain meds
disorient people to place and circumstance. *Where am I?*
What happened to me? . . . Oh . . . yeah, I had surgery.

The patient moves and is startled by intense pain. They
hold still and note the pain diminishing. That makes them
cautious about additional movement. But people aren't
used to staying perfectly still and move again. That triggers
another spasm of pain. *Ahh, this is awful. It hurts way more*
than I thought it would. From then on, the patient moves
slowly and carefully, trying to minimize the agony even
the slightest movement triggers.

The amount of hurt varies with the operation. Large
incisions in the upper abdomen and the side of the chest
are the worst. Breathing causes motion at the site of those
cuts, making it impossible to avoid pain by staying still.
An incision at the center of the chest moves less with each
breath than those on the side, but the central incision for

open-heart surgery has a broken bone under it, adding to the pain.

Many factors contribute to the amount of pain post-op patients experience. Sometimes treatment requires so much narcotic that the person falls asleep. That carries its own set of dangers, from shallow breathing increasing the risk of pneumonia to clots forming in the legs from lack of movement. The variety of operations and the range of experiences are vast, but many patients are unpleasantly surprised, at least briefly, by the degree of suffering they experience.

However, recent advances have significantly reduced post-op pain. The techniques include a variety of nerve blocks with local anesthetics, injected by the surgeon while the wound is open or by an anesthesiologist using ultrasound to locate the exact place where the medicine needs to be put for best effect. The introduction of minimally invasive surgery has also significantly reduced post-op pain. This requires video game–style skills using tiny scopes and instruments inserted deep into the body. Whereas a gallbladder operation once started with a six-inch incision in the right upper abdomen, surgeons can now remove that organ laparoscopically using three or four tiny cuts (around 0.2 to 0.4 inches long) resulting in much less post-op pain. Thoracoscopic surgery has similarly transformed operations on lungs. Arthroscopic surgery has done the same for orthopedic procedures on shoulders, hips, and knees.

Nonetheless, despite these advances, pain continues to bedevil recovery. We do our best to deal with it. Our best today is far better than it was just a few years ago, but we still have a long way to go.

Pain has a protective function, warning us not to do something that might cause harm: don't touch a hot stove to avoid burn injury; don't move in a way that puts traction on your surgical wound and retards healing. A rare and dangerous genetic abnormality causes insensitivity to pain. People with this condition suffer cuts, burns, and other injuries made worse by their inability to feel pain and take steps to avoid harm. This can result in severe injuries, including wounds to feet and hands that can result in amputations. They can chew their tongue, cheeks, and lips unaware of self-mutilation in real time. Most of these people die prematurely, often before age 25.[1]

While we can be thankful for the ability to feel pain, too much of this good thing can be horrible. A lot of post-surgical pain just reminds you that your body has suffered trauma. Big surgery is big trauma and big trauma tends to cause big pain. As an anesthesiologist and a human being, I am all in for the alleviation of big pain.

The first thing I remember after my operation was waking up in the cardiac surgery ICU and feeling like a dragon had scorched the center of my chest and stomped on it. My upper body felt as if it were on fire when I lay still. Movement only made things worse—much worse. This pain was clearly different from the exercise-induced burning before surgery, more intense and closer to the surface, mainly the result of my sawed-in-half breastbone.

When I first opened my eyes that morning, I saw Rachel sitting by my bedside, looking like a beautiful guardian angel. Weeks later, she told me that she had made an extra effort to look her best. Every day I was in the hospital, she wore pretty dresses and makeup—part of her effort to help raise my spirits. As I opened my eyes and caught my first glimpse of Rachel, I smiled weakly. She leaned forward, reached for my hand, flashed a radiant smile, and went through the motions of our secret "I love you" signal.

The day passed for me in a narcotic haze. I drifted in and out of awareness and remember only intermittent fragments: walking around the ICU; Rachel squeezing my hand to comfort me. Every time I woke up, I felt intense pain in the center of my chest, and every time I moved while asleep, I woke up.

The movement of my chest caused pain with every breath, both on inspiration and expiration. Deep breaths hurt even more. Shallow inspiration, the instinctive response to reduce pain, results in deflated air sacs in the lungs—a condition called *atelectasis*—and less efficient ventilation. It can eventually lead to pneumonia. Getting out of bed and walking stimulates deeper breathing and helps prevent respiratory problems.

Muscle movement while walking squeezes the veins in the legs and propels blood up toward the heart. That keeps blood from remaining stagnant in the lower extremities and helps prevent clot formation. Such clots can migrate through the heart and into the lungs, and can block circulation in one of its arteries. If this happens, it's called a *pulmonary embolus*. Pulmonary emboli can cause shortness of breath, coughing, profuse sweating, clammy skin, and sharp pain in the chest and arms—similar to the symptoms of a heart attack. A large enough pulmonary embolus can be fatal.

I was groggy when my nurse first came into my room. He flashed a warm smile and asked, "Do you feel ready to take a walk?"

I said, "Yes."

It wasn't true. I would have preferred to lie motionless to minimize the pain, but I was determined to do everything in my power to get well as quickly as possible. Besides, this nurse was bursting with enthusiasm. I felt he would provide me with good support to get moving.

The several IV bags, chest tubes, and monitors attached to me made getting out of bed a cumbersome maneuver. The nurse gently placed his arm under my back and helped me sit up. I gingerly worked my body around wires and tubes, dangled my feet over the side of the bed and stood up. The nurse picked up my chest tube drainage container in his left hand, pushed my wheeled IV pole with his left arm, and steadied me with his right arm. He did this with practiced dexterity, like a skilled waiter smoothly navigating narrow corridors between restaurant tables while balancing multiple dishes, making it all look easy. With Rachel on my right and the nurse on my left, we inched out of the room.

The center of my chest hurt, especially when I pulled my shoulders back, not wanting to walk like a hunched old man. The pain and the concern that stretching my incision that way might slow healing kept me from doing it too much.

We completed one circle around the ICU, a distance of about 50 yards. At the door to my room, the nurse asked, "Do you want to go back to bed?"

Hell yes, I thought silently, but aloud I said, "Nope, I can go around again."

I felt tired even before we began but grimly pushed forward. I rejected the offer to stop after the second lap as well. My determination to do everything within my power to promote swift and full recovery motivated my every slow, laborious step. We finished three circles around the ICU before I collapsed back into bed.

I thought this was still the day of my operation until Rachel informed me otherwise. I had been unaware that an afternoon and a night had come and gone.

A couple of hours after my walk, near noon the day after my surgery (post-operative day 1), Amy Palmer, a cardiac surgery physician assistant, came in to remove two of my chest tubes. The maximum amount of postsurgical oozing and bleeding takes place in the initial hours after an operation. On subsequent days, a smaller number of drains can adequately siphon excess fluid away from the wound. Surgeons take drains out sequentially as the fluid collected from them decreases.

"This will hurt for just a second. Take a deep breath and hold it," Amy instructed.

When a chest tube is pulled out, air can enter through the hole and compress the lungs and heart. By taking a deep breath before a tube is removed, you prevent air from rushing into the thoracic cavity through the chest tube hole. As Amy yanked out the first drainage tube, I felt a sharp stabbing pain. Just as she had promised, it quickly went away.

Many minor procedures hurt intensely, even if only briefly. People can endure it; they must endure it. There is no getting around the fact that removing a chest tube hurts. General anesthesia could eliminate the suffering completely, but administering that at the bedside for something so fleeting would entail more danger and effort than it's worth. Patients can also receive a narcotic pain medicine prior to such procedures. That reduces "discomfort," medicine's standard euphemism for pain, but not without the side effects of drowsiness and a reduction in the rate and depth of breathing. Narcotics can also cause nausea and constipation.

Each time I've been a patient since becoming a doctor, I have been surprised at the intensity of pain and misery caused by procedures we think of as routine. It has helped me appreciate just how much we ask of our patients—how much we *have* to ask of our patients—and the amount they suffer as a result.

"Okay, you can breathe again," Amy said.

Sounds obvious, but doctors and other health providers need to remember to say that before their patients turn blue. Amy tightened a suture to close the tube's entry hole. She repeated the process with the second tube, and left two of the original four in place.

Every few hours, whenever I remembered, I used an incentive spirometer, a simple instrument designed to promote deeper breathing. The spirometer has Ping-Pong–style balls in four cylindrical chambers. Patients are instructed to exhale completely, then put their lips over the spirometer's mouthpiece and suck in as much air as they can. That action, done correctly, causes the balls to rise. A healthy person can easily lift all four. After an abdominal or chest incision, people often struggle to raise even one. Determined to avoid lung complications, I managed to push three balls to the top. I couldn't get the fourth to budge, no matter how hard I tried.

Later that afternoon, I felt ready for another walk, but getting up proved harder than I expected. In retrospect, the nurse helping me to a sitting position for the prior walk had made that task much easier. This time, I made the mistake of thinking I could sit up on my own. The effort increased my incisional pain, and I broke out in a cold sweat, with blood vessels bulging on my forehead. I fell back, totally exhausted but determined not to concede defeat. To reduce the pain of my next attempt to sit up, I asked my nurse for a narcotic and waited for the effect of the shot to kick in.

Fifteen minutes later, I tried to get out of bed again, this time with the help of my nurse. Pulling on his arm, I succeeded in reaching a seated position. From there, the walk went as before. Determined to make progress, I insisted on a full four circuits around the ICU before once again collapsing back in bed, tired but satisfied, proud of my accomplishment.

Small triumphs encourage us as we struggle to make tiny steps on the road to recovery. Getting out of bed with less help, walking a little farther, feeling a bit stronger, and every other sign of progress lifts the spirit. Each new success can motivate us to strive harder to make additional advances.

However, recovery doesn't always present as an uninterrupted set of steps forward. Setbacks along the way are common and can be most discouraging. To recuperate well, we need to keep a positive mindset and struggle on when complications arise.

Chapter 6

Adapt, Adapt, Adapt:
Navigating an Unfamiliar World

Everybody has a plan until they get punched
in the mouth.

—Mike Tyson

In the course of a serious illness, cardiac or any other type, expect the unexpected. We know what tends to happen and how long healing usually takes. But every patient's recuperation is unique and requires course adjustments to address its ups and downs. Not all steps of recovery are likely to go without a hitch.

Recuperating well from major surgery requires the right attitude. Smart patients take the steps most likely to produce a good outcome. They also put in the work necessary to promote recovery. That may involve getting out of bed to walk, even at the cost of pain and exhaustion.

In addition to working hard and making smart decisions, we need at least a bit of good luck for a good recovery.

Years ago, a physics Nobel Prize laureate giving an introductory talk to starting PhD students at University of California, Berkeley, stated that in order to do well as a physicist, you need to have three things going for you. First, you need to be very smart, but that's a given for anyone in that program. Second, you need to work very hard. That's a lot tougher because some in the group may not want to work so hard. And third, you need to be very, very lucky. This came from a man who had been that lucky, had achieved tremendous success, but recognized that even with an abundance of talent and a strong work ethic, all is not under your control. Even a smart, hardworking physics PhD can take the wrong path and spend years researching ideas that lead nowhere.

Writer and Nobel laureate Elie Wiesel was once asked what allowed him to survive Nazi concentration camps when so many others died. Wiesel gave a single-word reply: luck. He didn't want to give a different answer, because that would have implied that those who perished lacked the intelligence and will to survive. True, staying alive through Nazi oppression required having your wits about you and working hard to persevere another day, but many who met those conditions were killed just the same.

Emily Dickinson wrote, "Luck is not chance, it's toil." Acting with intelligence and working hard can go a long way to producing what looks like good luck. But sometimes the dealer gives the best poker player at the table poor cards. Much of life seems to depend on three crucial factors: optimizing what is under our control, acting smart, and working hard. That applies to patients, physicists, and everyone else. Do those three things. And then we may also need luck.

According to hospital lore, doctors are especially prone to encountering complications on the road to recovery.

Whenever a physician patient suffers a setback, it won't be long before somebody blurts out, "Of course: a doctor."

I hate that. Where does this notion come from anyway? Do doctors indeed suffer more complications than average? A corollary holds that doctors make lousy patients—that they don't follow their physician's advice, think they know better, and want to be in charge of their own care.

I intended to shatter this stereotype, to be a superstar patient, one who gets well faster than expected, just like all the injured gymnasts I knew back in college. Since inactivity after cardiac surgery can slow recovery and contribute to complications, I was determined to push myself to be optimally active.

I believed in following my doctors' directions. Of course, I expected them to explain what they wanted me to do and why, and I didn't hesitate to provide feedback to influence their recommendations along the way. In the end, however, I recognized that they were the experts in their specialties. My wisest course was to do exactly what they recommended. This is true nearly all the time for all patients.

If doctors or nurses deviate from standard practice in an attempt to go an extra mile for a colleague, they can end up doing more harm than good, fulfilling the expectation that doctors get excessive complications. Usual care becomes usual because it works best. After all, the goal is to produce the best outcome for every patient. Whenever something better comes along, it replaces the treatment that preceded it. This is the history of scientific medicine, with newer antibiotics, chemotherapies, and operations displacing older, less effective ones.

Any effort to do even better by doing something different than evidence-proven best treatment is likely to do the exact opposite. Celebrity medicine illustrates this phenomenon. People naturally assume movie and rock stars get the finest care. Of course they do—if they're satisfied with the same medical management everybody else receives. Celebrities who demand special treatment might get the care they want instead of the care they need. Elvis Presley and Michael Jackson got celebrity medicine, received what they asked for, including copious amounts of their drugs of choice. Smart patients prefer state-of-the-art, standard medicine.

When everything proceeds according to plan, CABG patients leave the cardiac surgery ICU on post-op day 1. I stayed in the CSICU until the third post-operative day. Despite my intention to disprove the stereotype, my hospital course reinforced the "doctors make problem patients" myth.

The evening after my surgery, my *central venous pressure* (CVP) declined—a sign of inadequate fluid in my vascular system. One of the primary reasons for inserting a CVP line is to monitor shifts in fluid status, which occur commonly during and after major surgery. Throughout the night, I received multiple doses of IV albumin, a plasma protein that helps increase CVP. My urinary output also slowed. The ICU doctors treated this with additional IV fluids and several doses of a diuretic (a drug that stimulates urination).

The most common reason for delay of discharge from the ICU after coronary artery bypass is an arrhythmia, and the most common arrhythmia after this surgery is *atrial fibrillation* (or a-fib). Anywhere from 10 to 65 percent of patients go into a-fib following an open-heart operation (different studies have produced that wide range of results). Giving a beta blocker before surgery, such as the metoprolol Dr. Drury had prescribed for me, reduces the risk. The most common time for the onset of a-fib after CABG is the second post-operative day.

With a-fib, instead of contracting in the normal coordinated manner, the individual muscle cells in the two upper chambers of the heart, the atria, each beat on their own. This transforms the atria into a quivering, chaotic mass that resembles a clump of intertwined worms, all wiggling in different directions. Blood still flows into the lower chambers, the ventricles, but with diminished efficiency. In addition, the normal pattern of each atrial beat followed by a ventricular contraction ceases. If it didn't, the ventricles would also quiver chaotically and blood would stop flowing to the brain and other vital organs, resulting in death. Ventricular fibrillation calls for immediate CPR, with the goal of restoring a life sustaining heart rhythm.

The excessive atrial activity during a-fib does trigger ventricular contractions, but at a variable rate, causing the ventricles to beat rapidly and irregularly. Some arrhythmias follow a consistent pattern. If a ventricular beat follows every other atrial beat, that's called a 2-to-1 block; if every third beat of the atrium produces one ventricular contraction, we designate it as a 3-to-1 block. Atrial fibrillation results in no regular pattern of ventricular beats. Doctors describe its pattern as irregularly irregular.

A little after 10:00 p.m. on November 5, 34 hours after the conclusion of my surgery and right on schedule for the most common time for this complication to occur, my heart went into atrial fibrillation with a ventricular response rate of 146 beats per minute. My ICU nurse saw this on the monitor and immediately informed the doctor on call. With the onset of a-fib, some patients notice their heart racing or feel faint, tired, and weak. Many others don't, especially when inactive. I joined the latter group. Commotion around my bed woke me up and made me aware that something was happening. Craning my neck around to see the monitor, I noted unhappily my rapid, chaotic heart rhythm. I wasn't afraid, perhaps because of sedation, maybe because I knew that this was not uncommon and would likely respond to treatment. However, I also realized, much to my chagrin, that my plans for an exemplary, swift, and problem-free recovery had already been derailed.

The ICU doctor on duty started me on medications with the goal of initially slowing down my ventricular rate and eventually ending the arrhythmia altogether. My heart speed declined promptly, and my atria returned to a normal rhythm within a few hours, before sunrise. Electrocardiograms prior to and after the episode of atrial fibrillation recorded my heart beating around 80 times per minute. I remained on medication to prevent the return of a-fib during the rest of my hospitalization and for several weeks afterward.

My arrhythmia never returned. Patients with no prior history of atrial fibrillation generally respond to medication when this rhythm disturbance follows cardiac surgery. Those who have additional reasons for a-fib tend to be more resistant to treatment. Risk factors include a prior history of a-fib, cardiac muscle abnormalities (*cardiomyopathy*), heart valve problems, inflammation of the sac around the heart (*pericarditis*), and alcoholism.

In response to the arrhythmia episode and my borderline low blood pressure, my doctors decided to keep me in the ICU for an additional day of close observation. This included another test, an echocardiogram, to measure the efficiency of my heart contractions and rule out the possibility of an abnormal fluid collection around either my heart or lungs. The test revealed nothing alarming, only normal heart function and no abnormal fluid accumulation anywhere.

Despite this, my feet looked purple and felt icy to Rachel on post-op day 2. When she massaged them, I smiled and said, "This is the best I've felt since surgery."

Rachel later told me her heart melted upon hearing that, but what I said was so true. I felt pain in my chest and weak all over. Tied to tubes from above and below, my movement was awkward and restricted. I struggled to swallow anything. My attempts at eating even soft foods resulted in coughing and gagging. Rachel massaging my feet gave me the first sensation of pleasure since surgery. I was ever so grateful for it. If I had the energy, I would surely have kissed her.

I went on two walks on post-op day 2, just like the previous day, still assisted by a nurse and my wife. In the morning, I trudged around the ICU five times. In the afternoon, our hike extended farther, into the corridor outside the unit. The going was still arduous, but my mood was lifted by my ability to cover more ground with slightly less struggle than the day before.

By the next morning—post-op day 3—with no further complications to my recovery, my doctors felt ready to discharge me from the ICU to the cardiac surgery post-operative floor. Before the transfer, they took out my central venous line and the urinary catheter. My arterial line had been removed the prior day. I interpreted the removal of each tube as another step on the road to recovery. Having my body relieved of some of its restrictive attachments felt liberating, but only to a limited extent given how painful my chest felt.

My ICU nurse and an orderly pushed my bed over the covered bridge connecting the building housing the CSICU to the main hospital. I had crossed this bridge on numerous occasions, by myself and with other doctors, nurses, and orderlies—pushing a gurney, ventilating a still-intubated patient after a major operation, monitoring their electrocardiogram and pulse oximeter tracings, or visiting one of my patients post-op. However, I had never before made this journey in a supine position with someone else minding the monitors. A few days earlier, that would have seemed bizarre to me. By now, however, I had become accustomed to my role as a patient and just felt happy to be leaving the ICU.

My new room, slightly larger and far more private, contained a patient bed, several chairs, a continuous electrocardiogram monitor, a computer terminal for doctors and nurses to check lab reports, and a white bulletin board. Instead of a clear plastic wall and an oversized sliding glass door, only a standard, four-foot-wide wooden door connected this room to the outside. An adjacent private bathroom held a sink, a toilet, and a shower.

Inna, the licensed vocational nurse assigned to care for me, wrote my name and the date on the bulletin board. When she offered to wash my hair and back, I was reluctant at first, apprehensive about getting my dressings and incisions wet. But Inna talked me into it. I sat on a white plastic stool and leaned over the sink while she shampooed my hair. Immediately afterward, I felt refreshed, rejuvenated, clean, and more on the road to recovery. I was grateful for Inna's insistence and her kindness.

That afternoon, a 30-something physical therapist, dressed immaculately and looking athletic in all-white pants, polo shirt, and tennis shoes, came by. We walked up and down the corridor and a few stairs.

To my surprise, I graduated from hospital-based physical therapy within a half hour. "You can get around the hospital and can do everything you need to do to get around your home. You don't need any more help from me," the therapist chirped.

Really? That's it? That's all the physical therapy I get?

Of course, I was proud to so quickly reach a level where the therapist didn't think I needed any more help. At the same time, I had hoped for more coaching to regain my strength faster and get back to normal, not just to barely functional. Apparently, the goal of post-cardiac surgery physical therapy is rather modest, just enough to get by. I reached that level three days after surgery, while still feeling abysmally weak. *Mr. Crispy All-White may think walking up a few steps is enough, but that falls far short of my expectations.*

Rachel decided to spend that night in my room to see if she could help me in any way. Cedars provides a portable bed for a family member who wants to stay overnight with a patient. It consists of a metal frame with horizontal springs, topped by a thin mattress. Due to constraints of space and for ease of transport, these cots are narrow, lightweight, and not very comfortable.

With the interruptions from nurses checking my vital signs, a lab tech drawing blood before dawn, noise from activities outside my room and the quality of her bed, she didn't get much sleep. I did considerably better, helped along by a sleep-inducing pain injection. We both concluded it would be wiser for Rachel to go home and get more sleep on subsequent nights.

A loved one's illness causes stress, often lots of it. Worry and anxiety may be impossible to evade, but caregivers should make an effort to avoid exhaustion. Think of it as a marathon, not a sprint.

Using up too much energy at the start can lead to fatigue before the race is half over. Spouses often want to show love and devotion, to live up to the marriage vow "to have and to hold . . . in sickness and in health," but they also need to take care of themselves. Rachel spending another sleepless night at the hospital would have been bad for both of us, since she would have been more tired and less able to aid me the next day.

The patient also has responsibilities to their spouse. They shouldn't make unreasonable demands on family members and friends. Doing so may breed resentment.

When both members of a couple act with understanding and compassion, an illness can bring them closer, strengthen the bonds of love by going through tribulations together.

The stresses of caregiving increase with time. Those looking after someone with a chronic condition such as paraplegia or dementia frequently develop "caretaker stress syndrome," characterized by physical, mental, and emotional exhaustion. Symptoms include anxiety, mood swings, sleep disturbance, resentment, and depression. Lab tests show increased levels of stress hormones and lowered immune response.

A marathon has a clearly defined length, 26.2 miles. Major illness is all the more stressful for caretakers because the duration of recovery is variable. The endpoint may shift and cause mounting frustration.

Chapter 7

Enduring Discomfort:
Building Resilience in Recovery

> Mama always said life was like a box of choco-
> lates. You never know what you're gonna get.
>
> —from *Forrest Gump*,
> a novel by Winston Groom
> (better known from the movie)

Former Secretary of Defense Donald Rumsfeld famously said that there are "known unknowns; that is to say we know there are some things we do not know. But there are also unknown unknowns—the ones we don't know we don't know."

Known unknowns for a surgical patient are all the complications the patient knows can occur. What remains unknown are which ones and to what degree any of these potential complications will affect the patient. That only gets revealed in real time, but their occurrence doesn't surprise. Unknown unknowns are the misfortunes patients were unaware were even a possibility before getting clobbered by them. Blindsided by an unanticipated complication naturally feels more jarring and disturbing. The patient may wonder, *What else can happen that I don't know about?*

By post-op days three and four, my pain had subsided to an intermittent dull ache. Inability to eat then took center stage as my most disturbing symptom. Solids presented the greatest difficulty. I couldn't swallow fruit from an edible bouquet friends gave me and would surely have choked on anything from a box of chocolates. When I tried to swallow a bite of an egg-white omelet at breakfast, it got stuck in the back of my throat, inducing coughing and gagging. Every meal descended into an ugly and tortuous bout of choking, coughing, and retching, with tears streaming from my eyes and saliva mixed with bits of food dripping from my mouth. Sorry if this sounds nasty and disgusting. It was. By focusing intently, I could force tiny bits of softer foods like yogurt past my throat, but the effort was time-consuming and stressful. I struggled even to drink water. I knew I had to eat but dreaded the prospect of every upcoming meal. I had not expected this problem and was puzzled by it.

Pills, tablets, and capsules—oral medicines in all their varied forms—produced the greatest difficulty. While in the ICU, I had received drugs intravenously. Now I had to take oral versions of many of my medicines.

Prior to this, I never had a problem swallowing tablets, not even horse pills that cause many people to gag. Now however, a tablet of any size presented a major challenge. The magnitude of my struggle understandably correlated with the size of the pill. Contemplating the situation, I concluded that cutting the larger tablets in half, or even smaller chunks, would make the task easier.

During medical school and my surgery internship, I had acquired plenty of experience operating on people but none on pills. I operated on a tablet for the first time on post-op day 4. A registered nurse (RN) brought a handful of pills to me three times daily. I stared intently at the tablets and strategized over the sequence of cutting and swallowing. I would swallow a small tablet, then give my throat and nerves a bit of rest while bisecting a larger one. I alternated cutting and swallowing. Some gulps went well; others resulted in choking, coughing, and tears. To improve my prospects of getting all the medicine down, I chopped some of the submarine-shaped behemoths into three and four segments.

I complained about my swallowing distress to all my doctors. My symptoms were duly recorded in the chart, but that's as far as it went. Perhaps I didn't make the level of my despair clear enough. None of my doctors had visited during a mealtime ordeal and witnessed the full spectacle of its misery. Not knowing why I had this problem or what could be done about it left me feeling helpless and frustrated. By the afternoon of post-op day 4, after struggling to get down a few mouthfuls of mashed potatoes and several gulps of water for lunch, my desperation boiled over. I had to do something.

My intent from the start was to be a good patient, an easy patient, not someone who expects anything out of the ordinary. I was determined not to be a demanding patient, the kind that burdens the staff with unnecessary tasks.

When I was a medical student, a classmate and I heard a patient plead, "Please, someone please help me." She wasn't our patient, but we went into her room and asked what help she wanted.

"Please draw the curtain for me. It's too dark in here," she said. We did.

"No, that's too much. Now it's too light. Please close it a bit." We closed the curtain a couple of inches.

"No, that's too much. Open it a bit." After a couple of more adjustments by inches and finally fractions of inches, my classmate and I walked out. As we did, from the hallway, we heard again, "Someone please help me." This time we walked on. This is not an urban legend. It actually happened to me.

Similar things happen all the time. Some patients expect nurses to fluff their pillows repeatedly. Or want a grilled cheese sandwich delivered right away. "No, not American cheese. I want Swiss." Nurses don't have time for that. They have other patients with more pressing problems. They also can't get a doctor to materialize right away, unless the situation is a genuine emergency. Don't hesitate to ask when you have a need, but be reasonable. It sounds obvious, but not always to a sick people in distress that feels major to them.

My plan was to never make any unusual demands. But now—prior resolutions be damned—I was desperate enough to do whatever it took to resolve my swallowing problem.

A doctor might not visit me until the following morning—definitely not soon enough. I figured that I could ask my nurse to contact Dr. Drury or pick up the phone and call his office myself. This was a problem gastroenterologists treat, and Kevin would no doubt contact one for me. However, I knew many excellent gastroenterologists through my work in the GI Lab. *Why not just cut out a step and speed things up? What harm could there be in me calling a gastroenterologist to get advice?*

I picked up my bedside phone and rang Dr. Jeffrey Conklin. He had been my gastroenterologist four years earlier when I underwent a laparoscopic fundoplication, an operation to eliminate gastroesophageal reflux disease (GERD), my most serious surgery prior to the CABG.

That procedure consists of wrapping a small portion of the upper part of the stomach around the bottom end of the esophagus to reinforce the lower esophageal sphincter. A downside is that inflammation can cause food to hang-up at the entrance to the stomach for several days after surgery. Once the swelling subsides, this problem, along with the GERD, generally goes away. I experienced swallowing difficulties for the first few days after that operation, but they had faded into distant memory long before my hospitalization for heart surgery.

Jeff suggested getting a pair of diagnostic X-ray procedures—an *esophagram* and a video swallow study. However, he had answered my call just as he was about to walk out the door, drive to the airport, and leave town on vacation. He couldn't see me and make his flight.

While I was thinking about how to get the process moving quickly and diplomatically, Kevin came by. I explained to him what Jeff had recommended. He agreed with Jeff's plan and ordered the tests. I felt somewhat relieved, mainly by knowing my swallowing problem would be investigated, but also because Kevin didn't appear to mind my self-initiated consult.

The following morning, a technician transported me on a gurney to the ground-floor radiology suite. An excellent radiologist I had known for years and a speech therapist, Marietta Gold, whom I met there for the first time, supervised my procedures. We started with the esophagram. This diagnostic test begins with the patient swallowing a radio-opaque (visible on X-ray) solution. The radiologist then watches the progress of the fluid as it passes from the esophagus into the stomach while technicians film an X-ray movie of the event.

Sure enough, it revealed a slight narrowing of the esophagus. According to the report, "When the patient swallows in the horizontal position, there is likely to be incomplete emptying of the esophagus. This would be more prominent if the patient were taking solids such as tablets. These might wedge into the narrow lumen and act like a ball in a ball valve."

Of course, I hadn't been swallowing my meals and medicines in the horizontal position. I was struggling too hard to get anything down sitting straight up. If it would have helped, I would gladly have done all my swallowing standing up or in any contorted position my incisions allowed. Never mind. We now had a possible explanation for my difficulties, along with X-ray proof demonstrating the problem. Good news.

With a diagnosis established, the radiologist raised the possibility that we could stop the examination without the video swallow procedure, sparing me the further travail of having to battle to get a bunch of additional items down my throat. That sure sounded good to me, already frazzled from the struggle of swallowing the radio-opaque solution numerous times.

Marietta shot down that idea. She insisted we needed to do the video swallow to make sure nothing at the throat level was contributing to the problem. I listened intently to the discussion between the radiologist and the speech therapist, the former attempting to be kind and spare me further discomfort, the latter advocating for a more complete diagnostic workup. Subjecting me to an uncomfortable test would cause stress and distress. Diagnostic procedures can also lead to complications. And of course, additional testing meant additional expense to the hospital and a larger bill for the patient. Unless the second study was likely to produce useful information, it deserved to be cancelled.

Marietta argued that it could reveal an additional problem, and the radiologist soon agreed. Not examining all the anatomy involved in swallowing could lead to missing the real diagnosis, or at least to doubts about having missed it. Setting up the test at a later time to rule out a second problem would require much more effort than going ahead with everybody already in place and ready to proceed. Though stressed and fatigued, I also knew Marietta was right.

I faced a menacing army of six food-filled Dixie cups with grim determination. They stood in a straight line on the table in front of me, each holding a radio-opaque piece of food of a different consistency, ranging from pure liquid to custard to solid. My task was to swallow from each cup, one by one, while a video X-ray recorded the action in the back of my throat. The challenge reminded me of Japanese martial arts movies, where the hero faces a series of opponents, each of whom politely stands in line and waits his turn to fight a one-on-one battle, instead of all rushing him at once with overwhelming force.

As soon as the radiologist and Marietta looked at the first video swallow, I heard lively, excited chatter. They obviously saw something of interest. At their behest, I swallowed, or at least attempted to swallow successive slugs from the enemy cups. Placing a portion of the yogurt-consistency sample in my mouth, I tried to gulp it down on command. As we moved from one Dixie cup to the next, I alternately swallowed, gagged, and coughed. Despite the struggle involved, I was thrilled about the prospect of discovering the source of my problem, and hopefully a solution.

When a healthy person swallows, everything in the back of the throat goes down. In my case, only around half the food or liquid moved into my esophagus, while the rest remained pooled in the back of my throat. A second swallow cleared half of what was left behind and a third cleared half of what remained after the second. Quoting from the report, "Even after three swallows, there was still pooling in the pharynx. The patient was therefore breathing through a puddle of previously swallowed material."

In addition, "Pooling was least with thinner water-consistency boluses. There was more pharyngeal pooling with thicker consistencies, such as nectar and puree. We did not try solid foods." *Thank you for that bit of mercy.*

Marietta and the radiologist also made an additional significant discovery. The stuff I swallowed all went down on the left side of my esophagus, through the left lateral food channel. Normally, equal amounts go down the right and left sides. The lack of action on my right side indicated a right *pharyngeal palsy,* or muscle weakness. The portion destined for the right lateral food channel, instead of proceeding down remained in the back of my throat, causing the pooling.

Marietta asked me to swallow with my head turned to the right and then to the left. The pooling was lessened, and I felt more comfortable, with my head facing right. She instructed me to eat meals with my head turned that way.

I was ever so grateful to Marietta. Her insistence that we do the video swallow study led to discovering the true source of my problem and a strategy to reduce it. She was a star, the hero of that day.

The video swallow results got the attention of my doctors. Instead of just me complaining about my swallowing, we now had inscribed in my chart a genuine, objective-test-proven diagnosis: pharyngeal palsy. The simple act of writing a diagnosis on a medical record gives it extra gravitas and raises the urgency for resolution. It's much harder to ignore than a verbal complaint. Once it's in writing, a diagnosis calls for an explanation and treatment, if one is available.

Pharyngeal palsy means weakness or paralysis of muscles in the upper neck, the portion called the pharynx or throat. Naturally, I wanted to know whether this problem was a brief glitch or a lifelong curse.

Pharyngeal palsy falls into the T or throat part of the domain of ENT (ear, nose, and throat) specialists. At my request, Kevin contacted Martin Hopp, a very capable ENT doctor, also renowned for the mouthwatering chili he cooks for hospital potlucks.

Marty came by the next day. A jovial man, dark haired and tall, he was always full of empathy. He greeted me warmly. Marty sat down on the chair next to my bed, listened to my story, and examined my throat on the outside and inside. For the latter, he used a traditional doctor's concave head mirror, just like the one old-time country doctors wore.

Marty told me he had seen this problem numerous times after open-heart surgery. The cause is unknown, which invariably leads to competing speculative theories. Laryngoscopy and the endotracheal tube placement could irritate the throat. Since this symptom is more common after open-heart surgery than other operations requiring intubation, that cannot be the full explanation. Sternotomy, cutting and spreading of the breastbone, could cause swelling and other damage in the chest that somehow affects the swallowing process. There might be a central neurological source, some injury to a portion of the brain during bypass. The real cause could be any of these alone or in combination. It could also be something altogether different that we just don't know, either by itself or in combination with one or more of these suspected factors.

Whatever the cause, I most wanted to know the prospects for cure. Marty reassured me, "This problem goes away on its own. Usually takes a couple of weeks. I've never seen it last over a month. It's not fun. Actually, it's downright miserable." He ruefully shook his head and continued, "Sorry . . . but you just have to wait it out." Time—doctors often say "tincture of time," letting the body mobilize its own healing resources—is frequently all the medicine you need.

I felt much better after Marty's consultation. Prior to it, I had no idea when if ever this torment would cease. Assured of its limited duration, I could face my eating disability with less distress. I felt ready to combat my next meal . . . almost.

I routinely turned my head to the right while swallowing. By post-op day 6, I could finish a full container of yogurt, not with ease but by concentrating intently on each swallow. It might sound like a small triumph, but the progress boosted my confidence and my mood. I proudly told Rachel, "I dominate yogurt." Solids remained a nearly insurmountable challenge. By chewing soft foods into tiny morsels, taking my time, I could slowly eat small amounts. Each meal remained a prolonged, nasty ordeal.

Around this juncture, I made a surprising discovery. A spoonful of sugar may have been Mary Poppins' secret, but for me sparkling water helped the medicine go down. I had previously considered expensive bottled waters to be a brazen marketing scam, but at this time I temporarily became a fan of Perrier. I am not sure what mechanism was responsible, but it was also easier to swallow sparkling water than flat water to quench my thirst. Thereafter, Rachel kept the small refrigerator in my room well stocked with tiny bottles of Perrier.

After the mystery of an unknown unknown is converted to a known unknown, patients have a clearer understanding of their situation, which is often not as bad as their worst fears. With the cause of my swallowing problem now known, and Marty's confidence that the problem would go away within a month, I felt reassured and more optimistic. People can withstand misery with much greater ease when they know that it has an endpoint. Patients know from the start, or soon realize, that recuperating from a major operation is a long process and requires endurance.

Chapter 8

Perseverance Through Pain:
The Marathon of Healing

Pain is temporary, quitting lasts forever.

F aced with adversity, most of us draw upon past experiences for guidance. Prior triumphs, small and large,
provide inspiration. *I was able to overcome an obstacle then;
I can do it again.* That notion helps strengthen our resolve
and helps us avoid despair.[1] If we have used the memory
of a particular prior experience for motivation on previous
occasions, it's likely to be recalled again. Such memories
can become evergreens, conjured up repeatedly at times
of crisis.

I took two long walks on post-op day 4, one with Rachel
by my side and one on my own. Since I was no longer
attached to an IV bag, I could move about with greater
ease. My ongoing struggle to avoid hunching while walking increased the pain in the center of my chest.

Patient floors at Cedars-Sinai stretch nearly the length
of a football field. I trudged from one end to the other
and back several times during each outing. While going

the distance alone, pushing myself to keep walking, I had plenty of time for wandering thoughts. They drifted back to a previous test of perseverance, running cross-country in high school.

I entered my first long-distance race in tenth grade. Challenged by friends on the track team who insisted that "Gymnasts are strong, but they can't run," I decided to prove them wrong by joining the cross-country team during offseason for gymnastics.

After a few weeks of practice, we rode a bus to a community college campus for our first race. Several schools and around 100 runners took part. The course wound over two miles of dirt trails, and guys had given colorful names to the more memorable parts. The dreaded final steep incline before the road sloped downward to the end of the race had earned the name "Puke Hill."

Halfway through the course, many guys switched from running to walking. I initially resisted that temptation, but eventually fatigue got the better of me. I resumed running, but by then I was in the final bunch. Coming off Puke Hill, I had to sprint all out to avoid the humiliation of finishing dead last. I crossed the finish line just ahead of the final runner. Then I walked a few feet from the trail and threw up. I felt miserable, far more from my dismal performance than from the nausea and vomiting.

A week later, my team raced over the same course. Halfway through, I saw many guys walking and felt the urge to do likewise—but I had vowed never to do that again.

Keep going, I told myself. *It may hurt now, but think how much better you'll feel in just a few minutes if you keep running. Hang on. Keep running.*

I finished the race among the first half of the competitors. Afterward, I felt tired but gratified. I never walked again during a race, though I was tempted every time. My times improved steadily, and by the end of the season, I was finishing among the front quarter of runners.

I returned to gymnastics and didn't think about running for the rest of high school. Then, during finals week of my first term at UCLA, while studying hours on end for a physics exam, I felt tempted to shut my eyes. But as I sat at my desk ready to close the book, I recalled running cross-country and thought, *Keep going. It may hurt now but just think how much better you'll feel a short time later if you just keep going.* So, I plodded on and finished preparing for the exam.

After that, I likened studying during finals week to running cross-country. Cramming many hours at a stretch was definitely not my idea of a good time, but the rewards outweighed the pain.

From UCLA, I went to the Yale School of Medicine. Yale operated under the concept that its motivated medical students would benefit more if they studied for knowledge instead of written tests. (Anyone slacking off would be exposed during oral questioning in small-group seminars.) Our exam-free idyll ended abruptly at the end of the second year with Part 1 of the United States Medical Licensing Examination (USMLE), or National Boards. After no written tests for two years, that eight-hour exam loomed as a colossal challenge. Throughout a six-week study period, I concentrated on memorizing and rememorizing as much as possible from thousands of pages of text in all the preclinical subjects. A cross-country race had ended in minutes; studying for finals week at UCLA had lasted seven days; studying for National Boards was the longest marathon of my life up to that time. But by then I knew that "Pain is temporary, quitting lasts forever." I studied diligently to the last day.

After Yale, my UC, San Diego, surgery internship felt like a grueling yearlong marathon, a grinding test of stamina and determination. I had no choice. Finishing was an obligatory step to earning a license to practice medicine. While slogging through, I vowed to make it my last long-distance race. Fortunately, my next stop, a residency in anesthesiology at Stanford, felt more like a fun run. After that, I plunged into a residency program at Harvard's Massachusetts General Hospital that sometimes felt like another cross-country ordeal. By then, however, I was determined to become an anesthesiologist and the finish line was near.

After completing all those years of schooling, more than eleven following high school, I felt that my long-distance running days were over, that I'd earned the right to live life at a comfortable pace. Of course, that proved to be naive.

In subsequent years, I've come to realize that life consists of a series of cross-country races. We have to push ourselves to run on numerous occasions when walking seems far more enticing. I don't ever want to let myself down by succumbing to the temptation to take a more comfortable route that inevitably leads to a worse result.

In recent years, I've returned to actual running—not just the metaphorical kind—and have entered several dozen 10Ks around Los Angeles. During those runs, I've watched others walk portions of each course, but I've never joined them, no matter how tired I felt. I couldn't have enjoyed the energy bars and the festive atmosphere at the finish line if I did.

My long-distance race after heart surgery included literally putting one foot in front of the other. Puke Hill be damned, I had no intention of slowing down to momentarily feel a little better.

As the days went by and I felt stronger, Rachel and I trekked hand in hand over different floors and corridors throughout the hospital.

Cedars' principal buildings occupy five square blocks of prime real estate adjacent to Beverly Hills. Due to the hospital's location, reputation, and broad range of capabilities, a large number of Hollywood stars and other celebrities choose it for their medical needs. The vast majority of our patients have nothing to do with making movies or recording music, but with a history of treating entertainers such as Marilyn Monroe, Elizabeth Taylor, Frank Sinatra, Johnny Carson, Michael Jackson, and Madonna, Cedars has earned a reputation as "the Hospital of the Stars."

Doctors who've worked at Cedars also comprise a distinguished list. They've pioneered methods of treating heart failure and brain tumors, techniques of minimally invasive surgery, and a host of other diagnostic and therapeutic procedures.

Bridges on several floors connect the original structure to a newer adjacent tower that contains 150 intensive care unit beds, all in private rooms. The bridges look futuristic, with floor-to-ceiling translucent walls. Going over them, staff and patients can see traffic and buildings around the hospital, including the fashionable Beverly Center shopping mall across the street. At night, the light from the bridges emits a dim yellow glow reminiscent of old London streetlamps.

Several times on our walks, Rachel told me how lonely she felt driving home each night to an empty and cold apartment. I tried to reassure her that we would soon be going home together. In reality, I didn't feel anywhere near ready for discharge. I still needed several doses of IV meds daily and was barely able to feed myself. Rachel and I both wondered just how soon my condition would improve enough for me to go home.

"I'm so looking forward to that day," she said.

"Me too."

On post-op day 10, proud of my increasing activity, I boasted to Amy, the cardiac surgery physician assistant, about my extensive journeys around the hospital. To my surprise, she was not at all pleased.

"You can't leave this floor. The monitors can only track you on 6 North."

Nurses on 6 Northwest monitor patients' heart rhythms to promptly detect changes that might require intervention. I had five ECG electrode pads stuck on my chest at all times. These were attached to wires leading to a portable telemetry unit that recorded my tracings and transmitted them to two screens, one inside my room and the other at the central nursing station. The wall of monitors at the central station reminded me of sport-betting lounges in Las Vegas casinos, except these screens were smaller and displayed the moving ECG pattern of every patient on 6 Northeast, instead of the changing odds on ball games and horse races. I imagined that both the casino and the hospital monitors were watched with equal vigilance.

While walking outside my room, I carried my telemetry unit, about the size of a television remote control, inside a pocket of my gown. Since I didn't recall anyone cautioning me about limiting my travels earlier, I had assumed the monitors could pick up signals from anywhere in the hospital. The nurses never came looking for me while I ventured to other floors. I'm therefore quite sure the monitors did detect signals from a far wider area than their home floor.

Sometimes patients hear doctors, nurses, or, in this case, a physician's assistant tell them something that doesn't ring true.

Telling me that the monitors couldn't detect anything away from the floor contradicted my experience. Saying so was on the tip of my tongue, but I held back. I felt that Amy would see it as a challenge to her authority, and as I said before, I wanted to be a cooperative patient. In this case, it wasn't very important to me, but other situations require clarification. For example, patients who doubt the importance of not eating before surgery definitely need to get an explanation that will get them to comply.

It also helps when medical personnel have accurate information. As such a person, I feel compelled to add that in nearly all cases, doctors and nurses do have the right information and patients should respect that.

Patients have the right to ask questions respectfully and get respectful explanations. Sometimes the discussions that follow lead to beneficial changes in treatment.

Good communication also requires perseverance and taking the long view. A quick admonition may be expedient, but in the long run, it can erode trust, which can affect patients' follow through. Similarly, patients who, for the sake of expediency or perhaps embarrassment, don't convey all their symptoms or the amount of alcohol they drink, substances they smoke, or past health issues, do a disservice to their goal of getting better. Patients and medical staff take the recovery journey together. Honesty and mutual trust facilitate achieving the best outcome.

Chapter 9

Small Pains, Big Gains:
The Lost Art of Patience

I've missed more than 9,000 shots in my career.

—Michael Jordan

O ne of the photos in the Cedars-Sinai art collection
depicts a bullfight. It shows a bull kicking up dust
while charging full speed at a matador. Four sharp barbed
sticks called banderillas, each about two feet long and decorated with multicolored streaming flags, dangle from the
bull's shoulders. The matador stands with his arms fully
outstretched above his head, ready to plunge two more
banderillas onto the back of the snorting, understandingly
angry bull. The most memorable part of the photo is its
title, "Now you're going to feel a little needle stick."

This picture has never been displayed in a public area,
just in a back room where only doctors, nurses, and technicians see it. Patients and their families don't need a
reminder about how some of our "little needle sticks" feel,
but it's something the doctors and nurses wielding those
needles need to remember.

Intravenous lines are usually started with a sharp metal needle that has a thin plastic tube (catheter) around it. After a needle is pushed through the skin and into a vein, the plastic tube is advanced into the vein past the tip of the metal needle and the needle is removed. The plastic catheter can then be connected to tubing that can deliver fluids and medication directly into the bloodstream. IVs are most commonly placed in the forearm and back of the hand.

Every IV line has to be removed eventually. The longevity of an IV line can vary, but sooner or later each line's tip will work its way through the vein wall. After the tip slips outside a vein, the fluid it carries oozes into *subcutaneous tissue*, the layer beneath the skin. If the process continues long enough, this fluid will produce a visible bump, which can be painful but goes down as the body gradually absorbs the liquid. The IV's puncture site through the skin also provides a point of entry for bacteria. Left in long enough, an intravenous line will become infected. IVs are therefore removed or replaced on a schedule designed to prevent these problems, usually within four days. Patients hospitalized for more days typically need to have repeat IV insertions.

The multichannel central venous pressure (CVP) catheter served as my main intravenous line during surgery. I also had a smaller IV in my left forearm, placed initially for the angiogram, the X-ray study performed the day before my operation. When the CVP came out, just prior to my transfer out of the ICU, the forearm line became my only IV. By the next day, it needed to be replaced.

A variety of personnel insert IVs, including floor nurses, IV Team nurses, and physicians. Out of all these groups, anesthesiologists are among the most skilled. When others have trouble placing an IV, they often call upon an anesthesiologist for help.

Every patient who comes under an anesthesiologist's care gets an IV, so we can give medication rapidly. I liken starting IVs to shooting baskets. If your goal is to get good at it and you practice a lot, chances are you'll become at least proficient—or you might blossom into a star. Nevertheless, even the best free throw shooter sometimes misses, and some IVs are more like three-pointers or half-court shots. People with large protruding veins provide the easy shots, the layups. Medical students develop their skills and gain confidence when allowed to practice on such juicy "garden hoses."

Like most anesthesiologists, I take pride in my ability to find veins even in the toughest patients—people with small fragile vessels and obese patients with hard-to-see, hard-to-feel deep veins. My strategy starts with warming-up these patients. One of the techniques the human body uses for temperature regulation is to dilate and constrict veins near the skin. When it's cold, those veins are constricted to reduce the volume of blood cooled by circulating near the surface of the body. When it's warm, these same veins dilate to help our bodies cool down. That's why veins tend to be more engorged and visible in summer heat than in wintertime.

People with large bulging veins are fortunate. They are likely to suffer fewer missed needle sticks, less pain and frustration. Young, healthy, muscular folks tend to have prominent veins. I advise patients with small veins to go to the gym and pump iron four to five hours every day for several years in order to develop muscles like Conan the

Barbarian, with their accompanying massive veins. Petite elderly ladies often chuckle as they promise to follow my prescription.

I was sitting up in bed at a 45-degree angle, with Rachel resting in a chair beside me when a nurse from the IV team arrived to start a new line around 5:00 p.m. on post-op day 4.

Before even putting the tourniquet on my left arm in preparation to insert a new IV, she declared, "Uh-oh, you have difficult veins."

I was shocked. As a former competitive gymnast, I have well-developed arm muscles and prominent veins. Looking at my arm, I noticed my veins didn't protrude as much as usual. Ironically, veins tend to be least prominent when people most need them to stand out. When someone hasn't had enough to eat and drink, veins become less visible due to dehydration. But my situation didn't look so bad to me. I pointed out a couple of possibilities to her.

"Oh, those are really small. I can give it a try here, but no promises."

I didn't reply. Maybe she was just setting herself up to be a hero when the needle popped into the vein lickety-split.

"Cleo" inserted a needle in my left forearm. I could feel her partially withdrawing and redirecting it a couple of times. Finally, she got a flash of blood but could not advance the plastic catheter. That meant that the tip of the needle had gone in the near side and out the far side of the vein. Cleo couldn't salvage the attempt, which is an outcome worse than missing the blood vessel altogether.

Puncturing a vein damages it and allows blood to seep out through the hole. Some of this bleeding will collect in the tissues surrounding the vein, forming a bruise. The body then has to absorb this abnormal collection of blood cells. That process can result in scarring the vein down, converting it from an open channel into a collapsed, useless bit of tissue.

The most effective way to prevent the destruction of a vein after a puncture is to hold pressure long enough for the hole to seal through clotting, thereby reducing the amount of blood leaking outside the vessel to a minimum. Busy nurses, doctors, and technicians often slap a Band-Aid over a puncture site after a few seconds of pressure. Knowing the value of easily accessible veins, after getting my own blood drawn, I always hold pressure for at least three minutes. Better to hold it unnecessarily long, which I probably do, than not long enough. Likewise, I try to make sure that my patients' veins are preserved and instruct them to hold pressure over their punctures.

Cleo decided to try my right forearm next and after redirecting the needle several times, got the same result. I wanted to be a model patient, one who cooperates fully and makes the job of his nurses and doctors easier. Despite my growing apprehension after two misses, I wanted to give Cleo the benefit of the doubt. *Come on. Third time has to be the charm*, I silently prayed.

Cleo went for a vein in the back of my right hand. She redirected the needle once, twice, three times. I glanced at Rachel and saw her leaning forward, teeth clenched, sitting on the edge of her chair, poised to jump up to save me.

The third needle stick hurt me more than the first two attempts. Why do some needle sticks hurt more than others? Of course, a larger needle cuts through more of the skin, makes a larger hole and understandably causes more pain. But same-size needles can feel quite different as well. Pain nerves in the skin are not evenly distributed and cannot be seen by the person starting an IV. Sometimes the needle enters as far away from the closest pain nerve as possible, and the patient feels little more than mild pressure. At other times, the needle enters right on top of a pain fiber and hurts more than usual. Some skin areas have more pain fibers than others. The inside of the wrist, just above the palm, tends to be more tender than the back of the hand.

We can inject local anesthetic to numb the skin. This is done with a smaller needle but the anesthetic stings as well. The tradeoff makes sense only if the IV needle used is large enough to produce more pain than the combination of the smaller needle and the local. The fluid of the local anesthetic solution can also distort the tissue and make it more difficult to find the vein.

The needle tip can also push a vein away, causing it to "roll." Having to advance the needle farther or redirecting it prolongs the procedure and causes more pain. Stretching the skin helps hold the vein in place, but often at the expense of compressing it, thus making it a smaller target. Experience and skill—and sometimes luck—enables an IV starter to hold just the right amount of traction to make the vein stay in place but not collapse.

Cleo finally hit pay dirt. Then she carefully and neatly taped the IV to my skin. On the tape, she wrote down the date, time, and size of the catheter, standard protocol for

IV nurses and useful information for anyone evaluating the functioning of the line later.

I felt sympathy for Cleo, a lukewarm amount to be sure after the mini torture session. But as somebody who has been on the other side, I felt Cleo's pain as well as my own. I was aware that her pride had suffered and that sometimes even the best free throw shooter misses the hoop.

Many months later, I talked about this IV experience with a friend of mine, a nurse who joined the IV Team subsequent to my hospitalization. She told me that Cleo is considered very skilled at her job. Too bad she had an off game at a bad time for me. My friend also suggested that knowing she was working on an anesthesiologist might have flustered Cleo. I don't know if that's true, but this is one situation in which being a doctor might have worked against me.

All sorts of fears loom over the patient experience.

One of my principal concerns going into surgery was the possibility of brain damage. How high was my risk? At one end of the spectrum, researchers have reported diminished brain function in more than half the patients a few days after bypass, with the majority of those subjects continuing to suffer at least some deficit five years later. Other studies found no long-term cognitive deficits.

Scientists have theorized a range of possible causes for these deficits, called *post-perfusion syndrome*, but the true reason remains unknown. Much of the speculation centers on the possibility that patients suffer tiny strokes during surgery. The most prominent theory postulates that small bits of debris, microscopic clots and air bubbles, enter the bloodstream from the bypass machine, travel to the brain, and cause these ministrokes. Cross clamping the aorta, a standard part of the operation, or other surgical trauma to arteries could also cause small bits of plaque inside those vessels to break off and end up in the brain, again resulting in small strokes. The blood that leaks into the surgical field, then gets suctioned off, cleansed, and returned to the patient to reduce the need for transfusion could also cause these events by introducing debris.

If the cause of post-perfusion syndrome is not ministrokes, or if it's not entirely due to ministrokes, the way the heart-lung machine pumps blood could be a culprit. Since the machine doesn't exactly replicate the way the heart propels blood, the rate and pressure with which blood reaches the brain could cause injury through some mechanism we don't yet understand.

Lack of understanding overall is the key to the problem. It's hard to reliably prevent a complication when you're not sure what's causing it.

Of course, statistics and theories produce thought-provoking medical literature, but for any given patient the only thing about a complication that really matters is whether it happens to them. I detected no obvious cognitive deficits during my first few days after surgery, but I also didn't test for any. Not yet. All along, however, I knew with trepidation that I would eventually have to do so for my peace of mind.

Awake at 3:00 a.m. on post-op day 5, flat on my back in the darkness of my hospital room, my mind restless, I sought reassurance by silently reviewing common drugs and dosages—sedatives, anesthetics, muscle relaxants, agents that lower and raise heart rate and blood pressure, rescue meds for heart rhythm irregularities. I reviewed drug after drug, several dozen in all, and felt a huge sense of relief as the numbers popped into my mind promptly, without hesitation, through many different scenarios, for patients young and old, healthy and sick.

To double-check my memory and thinking capacity, I multiplied a series of two-digit numbers in my head. For example, 96 times 52: 96 times 50 is half of 96 times 100 or half of 9600, which comes to 4800. That plus two times 96, or 192, adds up to 4992, the final result. I did this with several pairs of double-digit numbers. I felt no need to check myself on paper, which would have been difficult to do anyway, lying in a hospital bed in the dark of the night.

My informal test fell far short of a professional assessment of mental function, but I felt relieved. Elated. Other people might have recited the names of people in their high school class, or historical facts, or legal arguments, or conjugated verbs, or recited state capitals, or song lyrics. But listing drug names and doing multiplication in my head worked for me. By my estimation, my memory remained intact; my ability to think appeared to be unchanged; my brain was alright. Hallelujah!

I am quite sure I fell asleep with a hint of a smile on my face.

An illness subjects patients to repeated frustrations interrupted by smaller and larger triumphs indicating progress.

Conversely, we can interpret the exact same sequence of events as repeated successes interrupted by setbacks. Some of us are innately more optimistic than others, but maintaining a positive attitude promotes recovery. Sometimes a needle stick doesn't succeed. Then a short time later, we get encouraging news. This process conjures up fear and anxiety along with hope. Optimism battles despair as progress and setbacks fight it out throughout the recovery process. In most cases, optimism is warranted. Patients usually take several steps in the right direction for every reversal, and recovery beckons enticingly on the horizon.

Chapter 10

Unscripted: Handling the Surprises

It's always something—if it ain't one thing, it's another.

—Gilda Radner,
as Roseanne Roseannadanna
on *Saturday Night Live*

R ecovery from heart surgery, or any other operation, carries a known set of possible complications. What the patient and his or her doctors cannot know ahead of time is which ones will bedevil the recovery process and how severely. Sometimes one such complication rears its ugly head and becomes surprisingly troublesome, at least briefly.

The fact that a complication is known to occur after a procedure does not mean that we can accurately predict which patients will suffer from it. We can collect data on what percent of patients will have the complication, data on risk factors that make the problem more likely, but each patient is an individual and will react as one. Which patients will get a complication that occurs to say 20 percent of the whole group remains a known unknown until the problem reveals itself. The same complication can also present in a mild or severe manner.

A hiccup starts with the sudden, erratic contraction of the diaphragm and intercostal muscles (those between the ribs). This is followed immediately by closure of the vocal cords over the larynx. A rapid air rush into lungs elicits the "hic" sound.

A broad range of conditions can cause hiccups—anything that irritates a part of the anatomy involved in the "hiccup arc," including nerves and muscles in the chest and the section of the brain that sends signals to them.

I started hiccupping right after surgery. The spasms were a bit more annoying than a usual bout of hiccups, since every hic caused a jolt of pain from my chest incision, but they made only a minor contribution to my overall discomfort.

Amy, the physician assistant caring for Dr. Trento's post-op patients, explained that most commonly, irritation from chest tubes triggers post-cardiac-surgery hiccups. As the tubes come out, the problem typically goes away. My hiccups at that point were garden-variety, one every few seconds with runs lasting anywhere from two to five minutes. I went through several such episodes the first day and looked forward to having them stop once chest tubes were no longer inside me.

After Amy pulled out the first two drains on post-op day 1, contrary to her prediction, the hiccups became more frequent. She explained that this could be caused by irritation from the removal process itself. Manipulating one tube could also change the position of another, causing it to lie in a place where it aggravated the diaphragm or a nerve more.

During her rounds on post-op day 5, Amy observed the drainage from my chest tubes, saw a minimal amount of fluid coming out of one and a bit more from the other, the usual pattern when the body is healing from heart surgery without complications. She decided to remove the less productive drain. Again, contrary to expectations, the rate of my hiccups increased, this time dramatically, with three- to ten-minute sequences of hiccups occurring at least hourly. When I tried to eat, the hiccups on top of my swallowing difficulty made meals all the more agonizing.

Heading in the wrong direction worried me a bit, but I maintained hope that once the final chest tube was removed, my hiccup problem would end. That last drain had to have been the one in the most irritating position, and perhaps it had moved slightly to an even worse location when its companion tubes came out.

The remaining chest tube collected almost no fluid during the following night. So, on the morning of post-op day 6, Amy removed it.

There's an old story of a Dutch boy who held back a torrent by plugging a hole in the dike with one finger. That last chest tube, like that finger, had held back a massive flood. The hiccups that poured forth immediately after its removal were unlike anything I had ever experienced.

Each sequence began with a single hic, followed by another a few seconds later, and then a torrent, a blitz of dozens upon dozens of hic-bombs. After each relentless flurry, I was granted a few seconds of rest, just long enough for me to hope that the ordeal was over. Then the next round erupted. This went on and on, endlessly.

I was trapped in hiccup hell. According to Rachel, I even hiccupped while asleep.

During my first year in medical school, I had learned about the range of severity of hiccups. In most situations, they present as a self-limiting nuisance. At the other extreme, people have died from intractable hiccups that persisted for weeks, months, even years.

Charles Osborne, a farmer from Iowa, holds the record for the longest run of hiccups, 68 fitful years, from 1922 to 1990. That dubious achievement got him into the *Guinness Book of World Records*. He made guest appearances on *Ripley's Believe It or Not!* radio program and the *Tonight Show* with Johnny Carson. He even became the subject of a Bazooka Joe bubble gum wrapper. *Guinness* noted that Mr. Osborne's condition prevented him from keeping in his false teeth. He hiccupped up to 40 times per minute initially, then slowed to half that rate and eventually to once every 10 seconds, for an estimated total of over 430 million hiccups. Others have been clocked at as many as 50 hiccups per minute for weeks and months.

Mr. Osborne managed to breathe adequately throughout his years of affliction, but not everyone has been so lucky. If the hiccups are intense and frequent enough, the diaphragm muscle eventually fatigues and can no longer muster enough strength to keep breathing. The victim then needs to be placed on a ventilator to prevent death from respiratory failure.

Years ago, deadly hiccups seemed akin to an attack of killer tomatoes to me. At this point in time, however, I was no longer amused. A few hours into the ordeal, I began to wonder how long my hurricane-intensity hiccup storms could persist. I would have bet against my affliction lasting long enough to cause medical complications. However, I recalled the old Chinese proverb, "A journey of a thousand miles begins with a single step." It occurred to me that the ordeal of a million hiccups begins with the first despicable "hic."

I was miserable. There was nothing I wanted more than to stop those damn hiccups. It became my number one priority, my most immediate goal in life. I complained about them to every doctor that came to my room.

"I *hic*-need, some-*hic*-thing, for these-*hic*-hiccups-*hic* . . . *hic*."

People have devised a broad range of therapies for hiccups, mainly maneuvers that irritate the back of the throat. Swallowing crystalline sugar rapidly and stretching both arms overhead while swallowing vigorously are two popular cures I've recommended to my patients. But with my swallowing disorder, tiny sugar crystals melted in my mouth before going down. And because it would place tension on my incision, I was prohibited from raising my arms above my head.

With mechanical maneuvers out, we had to resort to medicines. There are many available. Like the mechanical methods, they all work some of the time; none work all the time. Therapy comes down to trial and error.

My doctors tried a few without success. On the evening of post-op day 7, Dr. Cheng, a gastroenterologist, prescribed baclofen, a medicine that acts by reducing all types spastic muscle movements.

Finally, after a day and a half of nearly nonstop hiccupping, relief arrived. I slept all night and remained groggy the next morning. Occasionally, I would still have a run of hiccups, but nothing like the torrential spasms of the previous day. Baclofen causes somnolence and the amount I received was making me too sleepy. I slept the entire morning, waking up intermittently to exchange a few words with Rachel, my nurses, or a doctor. Then I continued to sleep throughout the afternoon.

The gastrointestinal, or GI, team came to visit. Dr. Cheng was talking to me and my eyes kept closing. He stopped speaking midsentence. I told him to continue, that I was listening despite my closed eyes. He didn't appear to believe me. Rachel explained later that I had started snoring softly while he was speaking. I wasn't aware of that, and thought I'd heard every word he said.

The first priority had been to halt the attack of the killer hiccups. To take the best shot at that, the gastro-enterologist initially ordered a large dose of baclofen, 20 milligrams, three times a day. Having proved we could manage the problem with this medicine, we could now back down on the amount. He cut my dosage in half.

Around six hours after my first lowered dose, I suffered a run of hiccups. *Not again*, I thought, filled with renewed despair. I asked my nurse for an additional dose of baclofen. She told me that per my doctor's orders, I needed to wait two hours.

"Please call the doctor-*hic*-to change that order. My dose was-*hic*-reduced from 20 milligrams t.i.d. [medical shorthand for three times a day] to 10 milligrams t.i.d. because I-*hic*-was too sleepy. But if the 10 milligrams t.i.d. results in breakthrough hiccupping, I need to get more-*hic*-medicine sooner."

She made the call and after a bit of delay, I received my rescue dose of baclofen. The lesson here is that orders can be changed. If a medication doesn't produce the desired effect, a patient can and should ask whether a change can be made. Often it can, and when it can't, the patient should at least get an explanation of why not. Either way, the patient is likely to feel better, just as I did in this case.

Some patients might be reluctant to ask for changes in their medication, but they shouldn't be. They not only have the right to make requests, but medical care actually relies on such collaboration. Doctors and nurses use feedback from patients to customize and improve care.

When Dr. Cheng visited next, we discussed how to proceed. Thereafter, I had a standing order for 10 milligrams of baclofen three times a day, with an additional order for 10 milligrams up to three times daily as needed. I had the option of increasing my dose all the way up to the initial level. With this flexibility, I could titrate the balance between hiccups and sleepiness. The goal was to reduce the dose of baclofen over time, with the expectation that my tendency to hiccup would diminish in the coming days and weeks. As it did, I could eventually discontinue anti-hiccup medication altogether, probably after several weeks. I followed the prescribed pattern of dose reduction and suffered no recurrence of hiccups.

Even patients with no medical background can help facilitate their own care by actions such as moving from a bed to a gurney or, as previously noted, holding pressure over the site of a needle stick to stem their bleeding. Whenever I ask one of my patients to do something like that, I tell them, "There are no free rides at this hospital.

We put everybody to work." That generally gets a laugh and sparks a sense of camaraderie. We're a team working together toward a common goal. I think that's the best perspective, both for patients and medical personnel.

Doctors and nurses know more about medical conditions and procedures than the vast majority of patients, but every patient knows what he or she feels better than anyone else. The phrase "God helps those who help themselves," definitely applies to medical care. This time-tested sentiment can be traced back thousands of years, at least as far back as ancient Greece, when it appeared in Aesop's fables. Benjamin Franklin helped popularize this saying in America by printing it in *Poor Richard's Almanack* in 1733.

My IV served as a conduit for both medicines and fluids. The fluids helped keep me from becoming dehydrated, despite my swallowing disability. Some of the medicines gave me grief, particularly potassium.

Coronary bypass patients commonly receive potassium to prevent arrhythmias. Unfortunately, potassium hurts as it enters a peripheral vein. The faster it goes in, the more it stings. Slowing the rate of the drip reduces the pain but prolongs the process. So, my choice was between double the pain for half the time or half the pain for twice as long. I went back and forth on this a couple of times, hoping in vain that the alternative strategy would cause less misery, a classic "grass looks greener on the other side" illusion.

To prevent infection, I received IV antibiotic infusions several times a day. Some of these medicines also hurt, due to their acidity, alkalinity, or the chemical components of the drug itself. Patients often complain about this, but I had never previously experienced it firsthand. The pain can be reduced or eliminated by placing an IV in a larger or more central vein. By entering the greater volume stream of blood in a large vein, the offending chemicals are more quickly diluted and therefore produce less irritation. Of course, accessing such a vein presents its own set of difficulties and risks.

Irritation from potassium, antibiotics, and from the catheter itself can cause inflammation around an IV insertion site. Two days after Cleo placed an IV there, the back of my right hand glowed bright red and felt tender.

Over the ensuing days, the redness and tenderness on my right hand increased and extended. By post-op day 9, the vein inflammation, or *phlebitis*, involved a tract that went from the back of my hand to the inside of my forearm and just past my elbow. Although my arm was sore, swollen, and looked angry red, it wasn't among my top concerns. Pushing on the area of inflammation, I could feel tenderness only on the surface. The muscles of my forearm seemed unaffected. I felt quite certain that the problem was superficial. Hiccups and swallowing problems bothered me a whole lot more than my arm.

However, phlebitis as extensive as mine generally produces clotting inside the vein. Clots in a superficial vein don't tend to cause serious problems. Those in deep veins, however, can migrate toward the heart and then lodge in the lungs. This phenomenon, called a *pulmonary embolus* (PE), is a dangerous development that can result in serious respiratory and cardiac problems, even death.

Luminaries who've died from pulmonary emboli include Jimmy Stewart, the Oscar-winning star of *It's a Wonderful Life*, Mexican painter Frida Kahlo, and Kaiser Wilhelm II, the last German emperor. Rapper Heavy D not only died of a PE, he did so at Cedars-Sinai, one year after my hospitalization.

Phlebitis caused by an IV usually doesn't involve a deeper vein, but it can. If it does, anticoagulation may be in order to dissolve the clots and reduce the risk of additional ones forming. Dr. Drury ordered a vascular study, done at the bedside with a portable ultrasound machine, which generates high-frequency sound waves (ultrasound) to create images of blood vessels. It can show where blood is moving freely and where a clot has formed. My study revealed clotting in segments of superficial veins in my forearm and elbow, but not in the deep ones. My doctors prescribed low-dose aspirin, a mild anticoagulant.

That was ostensibly good news, yet I was still disappointed. My right arm *cephalic vein*, the large one inside my elbow commonly used for drawing blood, had turned into a hard, fibrous chord, no longer an open channel suitable for taking blood samples or starting an IV. Prior to this hospitalization, both my cephalic veins provided easy access. After phlebitis destroyed the one in my right arm, I was down to one usable cephalic vein.

This was a blow to my self-image. Since my high school days, when gymnastics practice added layers of muscle to my arms and chest, the condition of my body has been a source of pride for me. Until I turned 58,

I could boast of what doctors call a "virgin abdomen," one that had never been entered surgically. The operation to eliminate reflux ended that, but that laparoscopy left only a couple of tiny, barely visible scars. The incision down the center of my chest ended all pretense. And now, even my veins were betraying me. My once-fit body was losing its luster, taking a beating that couldn't be denied. As a hiccupping guy in a hospital bed, moving gingerly to keep pain down and running into complications, I realized I was no longer the exceptionally healthy dude I'd always been. Losing him was losing a part of my identity. The accumulation of setbacks during the course of my recovery were slowly pushing me to the unhappy realization that I wasn't ever going to be quite the same.

Illness tends to generate doubts about the future. *Will I be able to be my old self? How will this affect the rest of my life?*

This is particularly true when a disease or its treatment disfigures the patient. It could involve the amputation of a limb, an eye, or a breast. A facial injury can alter how someone looks and affect their sense of sexual attractiveness. These changes can affect our ability to perform on the job or engage in hobbies we enjoy.

One of my patients, a woman around thirty, loved to talk. She engaged in endless clever banter with her friends, and entertained her doctors with her wit and verbal agility. Unfortunately, she came to us with a malignancy in her tongue. "This is not the right cancer for me," she said. "Can you imagine me not able to talk?"

Uncertainties and changes in how we view ourselves or live our lives can lead to mental health challenges.

Illness and hospitalization, especially prolonged hospitalization, can precipitate feelings of hopelessness and
depression. We want to avoid these, but they are known
to happen to some patients and are therefore known
unknowns for any particular individual.

Chapter 11

Seeking Equilibrium:
Finding Balance in the Extremes

> So convenient a thing it is to be a reasonable
> creature, since it enables one to find or make
> a reason for everything one has a mind to do.
>
> —Benjamin Franklin

Upon receiving a serious diagnosis, many patients resolve to persevere—to overcome this challenge by doing everything humanly possible to promote their recovery. That initial bravado gets tested as the illness relentlessly wears people down over time, hour after hour, day after day, even year after year. Fatigue, pain, and setbacks accumulate to undermine confidence in a future worth the fight. Patients who admirably endure setbacks one, two, and three may reach an endpoint in their capacity to remain positive when complication number four clobbers them.

As previously noted, Mike Tyson observed that, "Everybody has a plan until they get punched in the face." Many can take the initial hits but eventually have their spirit and body knocked out by a relentless barrage that just keeps on coming . . . and coming. Doubt creeps in. Effort diminishes with exhaustion. Someone who initially surprised their physical therapist by how hard they tried can turn lackadaisical. A patient who has been following a medication regimen devotedly may start to slack off. Usually calm people may become prone to anger as their frustrations accumulate.

The sequential emergence of new annoyances and threatening symptoms builds up stress. That can erupt in senselessly lashing out at any available target—a family member, a nurse, the dietician who delivers a meal tray with white toast instead of wheat. That toast may be the proverbial straw that broke the camel's back.

No matter how tough a person may be, their limits can be reached. Some may crack in a few hours; others can endure for months or years. How long depends not only on the individual's innate fortitude but also on the duration and intensity of the pain, fatigue, and stress. A person with cancer may bravely withstand a strenuous regimen of chemotherapy but become too discouraged to participate with the same dedication when a subsequent recurrence calls for another round of toxic medication.

Studies have shown that a large number of hospitalized patients develop depression. It typically goes unrecognized and untreated and can lengthen their stays and lead to higher readmission rates.[1]

On the morning of post-op day 9, I noticed a new plastic band on my left wrist. I had received my first wristband, a clear one, on admission. It listed my name, date of birth and hospital number for identification. Everybody who checks into the hospital gets one of those.

Patients receive additional wristbands to alert the staff to potential problems. My second one, color-coded green, appropriately warned nurses and doctors of a possible difficulty with my intubation. (Placing a breathing tube in me is more difficult than average.)

But this third one, yellow, the color for "Fall Risk," caught me totally by surprise. *Outrageous!* was my reflexive reaction. Another in a growing list of assaults on my self-image. *I am not a fall risk. I am a gymnast with excellent balance! Someone snuck it on while I was asleep and unaware, unable to defend myself against this middle-of-the-night assault.*

I felt like Cool Hand Luke with three shackles around his ankles. I complained to my nurses, my guests, to everyone within earshot. "Who put this on me? Why? Look, I can stand on my left leg alone, also on my right. I can balance on my toes."

I demonstrated all three maneuvers to my two nurses. Both the registered nurse and the licensed vocational nurse (LVN) looked horrified.

"Don't. You could fall," warned the RN.

"Not a chance," I replied. "I am *not* a fall risk."

The yellow band caused no harm, except to my pride. It changed nothing. Neither my nurses nor my guests appeared to understand the intensity of my outrage.

In retrospect, I may have overreacted . . . a little. But being told that my balance was lacking struck a nerve. Hospitalized patients lose a lot of their identity, a lot of control over their lives. That yellow band felt like a gratuitous insult, a totally unnecessary attack on my capabilities. Just think of putting a wristband on a musician that declares them tone deaf.

I learned later that Cedars had initiated a program to reduce patient falls in response to a mandate from the Joint Commission on Accreditation of Healthcare Organizations. As a result, a much larger number of patients now receive a yellow wristband for more careful observation.

Caution sometimes calls for paying attention even to people at minimally increased risk, but precaution can be overdone. If too many people wear a warning band, staff may not pay special attention to the patients who truly present a fall risk.

I am aware that few patients would have reacted with so much outrage to a thin, lightweight yellow bracelet. Most probably wouldn't even know what it meant. Many wouldn't care. But to me, it felt like a stinging insult. And maybe the accumulation of pain and helplessness was by this time making me more sensitive and more prone to lash out over slights that under normal circumstances would just make me laugh.

That's what I wrote initially. Later, I found out that a then recently enacted policy dictated that all patients coming to the operating room wear yellow "Fall Risk" wristbands. Sedation and anesthesia cause unsteadiness. That's the logic behind placing such a warning on every patient in the preoperative suite. Of course, once sedation wears off, the warning ceases to be informative and can even become misleading.

I also realized I had mistakenly blamed a night nurse for something done by another person much earlier. I must not have noticed the yellow band during the initial days after my surgery. My anger was misdirected, both at that innocent nurse and her daytime colleague who refused to remove the wristband. The latter should have been made aware of the policy. Then she could have explained it to me and diffused my anger. With a minor change in policy and staff education, this whole conflict could have been promptly resolved with no hard feelings. And in retrospect, I could have felt less outraged by an inconsequential wrist attachment. The stresses of illness can make patients act in ways they typically would not— and may later regret.

Among the many medicines I struggled with, one tablet stood out as uniquely the most vexing and hardest to swallow: an inch-long, oblong monster containing potassium. The alternative route for getting potassium, by IV, was no longer a viable option since prior infusions of that chemical had most likely caused my phlebitis. So, I had to take this medicine by mouth or not at all. I chopped the behemoth into four parts and still struggled to finish off each segment, especially the two middle ones with sharp edges at both ends after the cutting. The tapered outer quarters slid down with slightly greater ease. I went after a middle segment first, followed with the two outer ones and finished off the final middle section last. The logic of my strategy went like this: start with a toughie while at my strongest, go for two easier pieces next, then rest a bit before the final challenge.

My potassium level on post-op day 9 came in at 4.1 (measured in millimoles per liter), near the middle of the normal range, which runs from 3.5 to 5.0. It seemed to me that my most menacing monster-sized pill might not even be necessary.

I asked about that when the cardiology fellow made his rounds late that morning. He explained that the potassium level can decline following cardiac surgery, something I already knew. He added that supplementation is routinely ordered to ensure it doesn't dip below the normal range (which can cause an arrhythmia).

"That sounds reasonable when taking the tablet doesn't pose a problem. But if the circumstances make taking potassium far harder, then shouldn't we re-examine the cost-benefit ratio?" I explained that I couldn't swallow normally, that downing this tablet was pure agony for me. "Is subjecting me to certain misery to prevent an unlikely occurrence really necessary? You have me on ECG monitoring at all times. We can promptly detect and treat any arrhythmias, and I haven't had any in days. Can we d/c [discontinue] the potassium unless my level gets too low?"

After a few seconds of hesitation, he said, "Yes. We can do that."

That's all it took. In less than a minute, he input the order to remove the largest, most dreaded blimp from my medicine menu.

I felt relieved. Rachel was astonished.

"I had no idea you can talk your way out of a pill you don't want," she said.

Since she hadn't worked in medicine, Rachel didn't know that patients negotiate with their doctors all the time. That can be good or bad. Sometimes patients argue against their best treatment and their doctors would be wrong to give in. But as noted before, patients can provide their doctors new information that leads to improvements in the quality of care.

When my doctors prescribed that potassium tablet, they didn't know just how much misery it would cause until they got feedback from me. That new information led to a beneficial change in my treatment. My potassium level never dipped below the normal range. I suffered no arrhythmias and avoided the agony of struggling further with the great white whale.

At that point, that bit of self-advocacy felt like a sig-nifigant victory.

I woke up on Sunday, post-op day 10, feeling much better. My hiccups were well controlled on a dose of medica-tion that allowed me to stay alert. Swallowing remained a problem, but my ability to do so was slowly improving. For the first time since surgery, I felt well enough to think about going home.

Except now another problem danced onto center stage—my white blood cell count. An elevated WBC count can be the first warning sign of an infection, but it can also be due to many other causes. Stress alone can raise white cell production. So can tissue damage and inflammation from an injury, including surgery. These causes don't require treatment beyond tincture of time, but a missed infection can be catastrophic. Elevated WBC levels therefore require ruling out an infection.

The normal WBC range extends from 4,000 to 11,000 cells per microliter of blood. On post-op day 3, my level came in at 7,400. From there, it increased daily and reached 19,400 by post-op day 7. That's when my doctors ordered an infectious disease workup. On that day, I was way too preoccupied with the attack of the killer hiccups to pay much attention to it.

To search for a suspected infection from an unknown source, doctors check for:

1. sepsis (bacteria in the bloodstream) with two blood cultures
2. respiratory infection with a sputum culture (mucus collected from the back of the throat)
3. urinary tract infection with a urinalysis.

My tests revealed no signs of bacteria in my blood, sputum, or urine. Nevertheless, my white count continued to rise. On post-op day 10, just when I was feeling so much better, it reached 24,600.

A rising white count, especially one that high, called for a repeat infectious disease workup. Of course, the most likely cause, my swollen right forearm, tender from phlebitis, was flashing a bright-red signal. But to make sure an *occult* infection (the term means *hidden*, and in no way casts blame on witches) was not brewing somewhere else, my doctors needed to again rule out infection in places it most commonly occurs.

I had no symptoms of a urinary tract infection—no frequency, urgency, or burning on urination. With no cough or breathing problems, my risk of a respiratory infection was also close to zero. And patients with sepsis tend to feel and look really sick. They often run a high fever. My temperature was normal, and, as noted, I was beginning to feel pretty good. In my evaluation, if any of the blood cultures came back positive, it would most likely be due to contamination of the culture, not sepsis.

Peeing in a cup for the urinalysis was easy enough. I had a harder time giving a sputum sample, since I wasn't coughing up anything. The meager sample I provided no doubt contained more saliva than mucus from my lungs. The blood cultures presented the greatest challenge. Because of the phlebitis, samples couldn't be drawn from my right arm. Each culture called for two tubes of blood taken either from separate sites or at two different times. Since bacteria might not be present in every blood draw, double sampling reduces the chance of missing an infection. On post-op day 7, the technician had extracted both specimens from the same place, my left cephalic vein, a half-hour apart.

During the second infectious disease workup, I dreaded being stuck twice. The chance of a positive yield on the repeat sample alone was very low. We already had two negative cultures from three days earlier and one new tube of blood to test. Besides, I simply felt too good to have sepsis.

"Do we really need to send another sample? It's going to be negative," I pleaded with the technician.

"Do you want to refuse the test?" she asked, sounding hopeful that I would.

My arm was tender, and technicians were having increasing difficulty getting samples from my one remaining cephalic vein. This technician had to redirect the needle to get the first sample. I felt that going through the pro-forma performance of a test that would almost certainly produce no useful result was not in my best interest.

"I guess so. If the infectious disease specialist really feels it needs to be done, we can talk about it."

So, for the first and only time during my hospitalization, to the relief of the person assigned the responsibility of getting the sample, I reluctantly and apologetically refused a test. Nurses must call the physician who ordered the study whenever that happens for any reason. If that doctor feels the procedure is important enough, he will talk to the patient about it. Nobody came to try to talk me into the additional blood culture. The third one came back negative, as did the urine and sputum tests. These results made me more certain of my working diagnosis for the most likely cause of the elevated WBC: phlebitis in my right forearm.

I felt pretty good the rest of the day. However just about any movement, even normal shifting of my position while sitting in bed, could trigger a brief burst of intense burning over the entire length of my sternum. Raising or lowering my chest between a horizontal and a vertical position caused pain that was much less intense than the first couple of days after surgery, and more fleeting, but still very unpleasant. Motion puts a strain on wounded tissue and initiates a pain impulse.

I strategized about how to minimize my pain before making any major move.

To sit up, I used the electrical controls of the bed to raise my chest from a flat to a nearly upright position. Moving passively eliminated the strain that accompanied the same action performed with my own muscles. Going from sitting to standing didn't require a change in the vertical alignment of my chest. That action therefore caused very little additional distress. I felt strong enough to go home.

The next day, my white blood cell count declined to 16,500, a step in the right direction but still too high for discharge. On the bulletin board in my room, the one with my name and the date inscribed on it, I scribbled on the bottom, "Number of days Kadar has been kept prisoner in room 6028." Next to it, I drew sets of four vertical lines and crosshatches, prison style, cheating just a little by including all the days since my admission for the angiogram. Perhaps a bit lame, but this was an attempt to inject a little humor to help diminish my disappointment.

I could check my lab results as soon as they became available by logging into Cedars' computer system with my password, using either the hospital computer in my room or my own laptop. I had done that several times during my hospitalization, whenever I wanted to follow my progress before my doctors had a chance to talk to me.

I accessed my medical chart through my staff portal, but all Cedars-Sinai patients can view their lab results through a different sign-in system. Besides reviewing lab entries, patients can use their computers to ask their doctors questions. This is particularly useful for those who are not hospitalized and have busy schedules. Of course, the amount of information any patient gleans from their chart depends on their ability to interpret what's there. A lay patient following the course of his or her white cell count could see it rising or declining as readily as I did. They could also read the interpretation of a chest X-ray or an ECG, but perhaps not understand it as well. So being a doctor does provide an advantage, but maybe not as much as you might imagine.

My infectious disease doctor, Phil Zakowski, assured me that if my white count declined as expected the next day, I could go home. A lower WBC level would signal that the process causing the elevation was resolving and therefore not due to a developing occult infection. The following morning, post-op day 12, I checked the results in the computer with high hopes. *Damn it.* My WBC count had gone the wrong way, back up to 17,900.

Phlebitis still remained the most likely cause, but a rising WBC count left room for doubt. My brain knew that my discharge was doomed, but my heart retained a modicum of hope. A short time later, Phil delivered the verdict.

"I don't feel comfortable sending you home with that white count, especially since it's higher than yesterday."

"Okay. I'm not happy about it, but I'll do what you think is best."

Going home with an unresolved issue can result in having to come back to the hospital a day or two later, much sicker. If I had a lurking infection, it could be detected and treated more promptly and effectively in the hospital. Since the infectious disease doc felt there was a significant enough chance of me having something that would need treatment, the wisest course was to stick around another day.

Nevertheless, I felt deflated. After two weeks in the hospital, I longed to go home. I missed my privacy, my own king-sized bed shared with my wife. I longed for the freedom to walk wherever and do whatever I wanted. After Phil left, I went over to the bulletin board and drew another vertical line on my prison-style calendar.

Amy came to check on me. I told her about how well I felt, even while going up two flights of stairs . . . *Oops.*

"Why did you go off the floor? The monitors can't track your heart rhythm. I told you before not to do that."

Okay, I was still in the hospital only because of the elevated white count. If it had come back lower, I would already be home, out of the range of in-hospital monitors. The risk of an arrhythmia was pretty low by now. Exploring wider made my walks more varied and interesting. However, rules are rules. Cardiac surgery post-op patients routinely stay on heart-rhythm monitoring until discharge. So according to protocol, Amy was right, even if it wasn't really all that important anymore. Nevertheless, I knew that contrition was my best course of action.

"Sorry. I felt so good, I forgot. But you're right. I'll stay on the floor today."

She scolded me again to make sure I got the point, and I apologized again. Then I stayed on the sixth floor for the rest of the day . . . mostly.

While in my room, I used my laptop to answer emails and to review my medical record. Rachel brought me the *Los Angeles Times* from home, and I read a few articles from it. I was getting ready to rejoin the world. Instead of focusing exclusively on my recuperation, I started to catch up on the news and resumed communicating with friends.

My prolonged stay initiated a visit from a hospitality nurse, whose job centers on making sure patients are pleased with their care. That involves both medical and comfort considerations. To help lift my spirits, she offered me a "special meal": filet mignon instead of ordinary hospital fare. With my swallowing problem, eating steak was out of the question, but I requested one for Rachel instead. She enjoyed the filet while I struggled with a soft bland hospital meal of some kind of pasta. I did, however, commandeer the cup of chocolate Häagen-Dazs off her tray. Although my primary motivation was the pleasure of tasting chocolate ice cream and I didn't think about anything more profound at the time, in retrospect, this minor act of rebellion was also an attempt to increase my autonomy, to make a decision about my life that the hospital wasn't permitting.

The hospital meal order sheets I filled out each day let me choose ice cream with lunch and dinner, but the only flavor available was vanilla. (At the time, I couldn't figure out what perverse reasoning made vanilla preferable to chocolate. Some months later, I learned the answer at an educational conference presented by a cardiac radiologist at the hospital—caffeine can alter the results of some heart X-ray studies. Because of that, coffee and tea, served almost everywhere else in the hospital, were banished from patient menus on the cardiac floors. Even chocolate, containing just a minute amount of caffeine, made the forbidden list. Since I didn't need any of the X-ray studies affected, my enjoyment of contraband ice cream caused no problems.) High-fat ice cream may not sound like the healthiest food for someone recuperating from heart surgery. But with my swallowing problem, I was unable to eat enough to maintain my weight. I needed calories, any kind of calories. And for the record, the chocolate Häagen-Dazs went down easy and tasted wonderful.

On admission to the hospital, I checked in at 132 pounds, an ideal weight for my five-foot-five-inch height. The day after surgery, the nurses recorded my weight at 136 pounds 10 ounces, but that included a couple of chest tubes and some excess retained fluid. I proceeded to lose a pound or more per day after that. By post-op day 12, my weight had declined to 124 pounds. My body was shedding muscle and fat at a rate that could slow healing and recuperation. If Häagen-Dazs produced calories I could swallow, then for the time being, rich, premium ice cream would be good for my health. At least that's how I explained it to Rachel.

My sleep pattern remained totally out of whack. I would wake up in the middle of the night from the pain caused by an inadvertent move in my sleep or from hospital noise. Sometimes, I just lay in bed thinking. I contemplated upcoming events: exercise for cardiac rehab and the obligatory time at home to heal. My mind also wandered in a random pattern to past events, often to times when I faced a struggle. *You've overcome challenges before; you can do it again.* A subconscious attempt to keep my spirits up may have been at work here.

The next morning, post-op day 13, my blood was drawn at six and the results came back three hours later. WBCs down to 15,600, the lowest count in over a week. After seeing the number on my computer, I wondered, *Will this be good enough?*

If an infection really was brewing, the WBC count would be expected to rise daily until treated. A declining level indicated that the situation was getting better. How much better did it need to be to reassure the infectious disease doc that sending me home was safe?

Phil came to my room a short while later and delivered his verdict. The trend had turned in the right direction— good enough for discharge. Hallelujah! Free to go home. No more hospital restrictions. The comforts of home. The joy of reaching a landmark in recovery. I was bursting with excitement.

While Rachel was en route to pick me up, I went down to the gift shop, no longer breaking rules by leaving the floor. My goal was to find a parting gift for the staff. I returned with a large box of See's gourmet chocolate, vanilla, and butterscotch lollipops, more than enough for everyone working on 6 Northeast that morning.

Rachel arrived. With my discharge papers signed, I still needed to go through the prescribed ritual for leaving the hospital. I had been walking throughout the building's hallways unassisted for days. However, newly discharged, I had to sit in a wheelchair to be escorted out. "We don't want any of our patients to fall and hurt themselves as they're leaving the hospital," was the explanation. This has to be a lawyer-mandated, cover-your-ass rule that nobody dares to question. One of the nurses gave me a parting gift, a pillow to place in front of my chest, to shield it from the pressure of seatbelts. As we rolled past the nursing station, lollipop-licking RNs and LVNs smiled, waved, and wished me well.

When a patient begins to feel better, hospital confinement can start to resemble imprisonment. You know it's in your best interest, but you just want out. You chafe at hospital rules that don't make sense in your case, or at least you think they don't. You long to regain greater control over your life.

Conversely, some people love to hang out at the hospital. Other than for occasional annoyances such as a needle stick or swallowing a bitter fluid for an X-ray study, a patient who feels good can enjoy a vacation from their usual cares. You get three warm meals a day and can ask for additional snacks. Nurses and aides attend to your comfort. You might meet other patients for engaging conversations. Visitors provide sympathy. Previously unmentioned complaints often pop up on the morning of discharge. Some patients can be hard to move out of the hospital.

Both groups of patients could be right. The transition home is a clear sign of progress, but like every stage in recovery, it comes with challenges.

PART III

HOME RECOVERY

Chapter 12

Home, Sweet Home:
Readjusting to the Familiar

There is no place like home.

—Dorothy,
in *The Wizard of Oz*

D ischarge from hospital punctuates a major milestone on the road to recovery. The patient gains the comforts of home but loses access to immediate medical care round the clock. Responsibility for help with mundane tasks shifts from hospital personnel to family. That can cause difficulties for people who live alone or with family members unable to provide the required support. It can also be physically and emotionally taxing for caretakers.

Some patients move to an assisted-care facility. Others hire live-in help or people who come daily to assist. The most ideal situation occurs when the patient has loved ones who are willing and capable of providing help with feeding, getting medicines from the pharmacy, other tasks required to facilitate recovery, and some all-important TLC. Some patients feel they have been discharged too soon, that they need to recuperate more to be ready for home care. Insurance coverage may dictate some discharges that feel premature.

What doesn't change at discharge is the attitude and effort needed for best recovery results. Patients have to continue their commitment to doing the work to promote recovery. As time passes, in most cases, that means increasing activity to get as close to pre-surgery normal as possible. What also doesn't change is the need to be considerate of caretakers: their job is difficult and deserves gratitude.

Fifteen days after I checked into the hospital for an angiogram and a probable overnight stay, I was finally out. With Rachel driving and the late-morning sun shining brightly overhead, we glided past buildings that appeared to stand out more clearly than usual. I saw sharp, crisp lines at their edges, reminiscent of an ultra-realistic acrylic painting. The familiar road home seemed more colorful, shining, and vibrant than on an ordinary day. I was elated to be cruising on city streets, free from hospital confinement, going home at last.

On Doheny Drive, we coasted past the Four Seasons, our wedding-night hotel. We turned right on Olympic Boulevard and rolled past the monument to the movie stars who in 1923 had helped preserve Beverly Hills as an independent city. Two blocks later, we passed Rodeo Drive, a little south of its elegant shops and the Beverly Wilshire Hotel, where the characters played by Richard Gere and Julia Roberts had occupied a suite in *Pretty Woman*. After Roxbury Park on our left, just past the high school, we arrived in Century City and then at the entrance gates to our condo complex.

I was invigorated by seeing my familiar neighborhood and glad to be home. Rachel drove into our building's indoor parking lot. We walked up the two steps to the lobby, took the elevator to our floor, and entered our home. My first glance past the entry fell upon the dining table piled high with several stacks of mail. I walked slowly from room to room, happily reacquainting myself with my home. I surveyed the furniture, my bookshelves, and stepped out on the balcony from the living room to admire the gardens below.

In the master bathroom, I reviewed my discharge instructions—eleven different meds, a total of sixteeen pills daily, seven in the morning, three midday, and six before bed. My prescriptions included one tablet to prevent atrial fibrillation; two to lower my blood pressure, one of which also decreases heart rate; a mild blood thinner; two to lower cholesterol; two to reduce stomach acidity to decrease the risk of an ulcer (often given as a precautionary measure after major surgery); baclofen to prevent hiccups; and an antibiotic. That's a lot of pills, but not an unusual number for a patient immediately after major surgery.

After Rachel brought home the haul from our local pharmacy, I arranged the plastic medicine bottles into straight, military-like columns. The whole collection consisted of five different sections, perfectly organized for easy access and no mistakes: four cylinders of morning-only drugs in the back row, a solitary noon med in the middle, three evening-only containers in front, and the two three-times-per-day and the solitary twice-daily meds in two columns of their own off to one side.

It didn't take long for military discipline to break down. The cylinders were out of formation by the next morning. I had to double-check the list three times daily to be sure of taking all the meds at the right time. Accomplishing that task required more effort than I had appreciated, giving me newfound sympathy for people who must struggle with complex daily medicine routines.

I spent that first afternoon home sorting mail, scanning articles from professional journals and magazines that had arrived during my absence, and chatting with Rachel. My activities resembled those of someone coming home after a trip of a couple of weeks, catching up on what had been neglected in my absence. Through it all, I felt exhilarated, positive, and upbeat, happy to be home with no monitoring patches on my chest, no vital sign checks, no longer hospitalized. However, my chest incision intermittently reminded me with brief spasms of sharp pain that the healing process had a long, long way to go.

Recuperation after heart surgery proceeds gradually. The sternum needs to heal like any other broken bone. That takes around 12 weeks. By then, most patients have recovered to the point of being able to engage in light activities and return to work, except to jobs that involve strenuous physical exertion. Those may require recuperating for as long as six months.

For dinner that evening, Rachel prepared leek potato soup, soft enough for me to swallow, yet more appetizing than anything the hospital kitchen had offered. Rachel had set a goal for herself to help me get well and feel better by preparing tasty, nutritious meals. She got off to a flying start with that soup.

I went to bed at 10:00 p.m. with Rachel beside me. We lay side by side, holding hands but carefully avoiding any contact with my chest. Nevertheless, our closeness and our hand squeezes made me feel loved and even happier to be home. Rachel promptly fell asleep, but I remained wide awake. After lying in bed for a half hour, I got up, went to my office, and read until fatigue set in. Returning to bed just after midnight, I lay down on my back and tried to sleep. This time it worked, until I awoke in the dark, peeked over to my left at the bedside clock and noted the time: 2:38 a.m.—not even close to a full night's sleep. My sleep pattern didn't appear to have benefited one bit by my more comfortable bed and surroundings. My biological clock was broken by the trauma of surgery and needed more time to heal and recalibrate.

I listened to Rachel's breathing, noting how it went from inaudible to audible and back to inaudible again. I was drowsy but couldn't get back to sleep. After lying in bed for nearly an hour, I went to my office, checked emails, and started picking my way through the accumulated backlog. When that began to feel tedious, I switched to playing *Snood*, an addictive computer game.

Around 5:00 a.m., I walked into the kitchen and ate a bowl of Froot Loops. To make the cereal easier to swallow, I let it soak in the milk long enough for it to become soft and mushy, not my normal preference. The rest of the morning, I read the newspaper and erased emails by inches.

Later that day I took a stroll around the grounds of our condo complex with Rachel. The complex is an island of tranquility in the middle of a busy metropolis—a quiet, gated, garden-landscaped enclave of six buildings. We stopped by the community's office. Tina, one of the secretaries, greeted us with a big, warm smile, "I was very sorry to hear about your illness, Dr. Kadar, and so surprised. If there is anything I can do for you, please don't hesitate."

She informed me that seven to eight times around the path inside the complex added up to one mile. That gave me a gauge to measure the quantity of my exercise. I walked at least one mile twice daily thereafter. My path frequently took me past retired folks resting on benches. For the first couple of days, Rachel occasionally asked me if I wanted to sit on a bench. I never did. A habit learned from high school cross-country: I never stop before the finish line.

Early in the afternoon, Rachel and I made an excursion to a supermarket a few blocks away. Then I needed to lie down and rest. My energy level was that low. A couple of hours later, one of my friends came by for a visit. We had a pleasant chat until I felt tired again. I rested in bed until the UCLA–Washington football game started.

After watching the game, I didn't feel sleepy, just tired. Rachel and I chatted in bed for nearly two hours before I turned on my right side and began to doze off. *Wait a minute. On to my right side? Wow! Another step forward—able to lie on my side comfortably for the first time since surgery. Yeah baby!*

I woke up at 1:30 a.m. and felt moisture over my chest and back, then a cold sensation on top of my shoulders. Night sweats! Heart surgery disrupts the body's thermostat. This commonly causes excessive sweating during the first few weeks of recuperation, especially at night.

I searched for my nurse call button before realizing I was no longer in the hospital. My T-shirt was drenched. Rachel had told me to wake her anytime I needed help, but I didn't want to bother her. Instead, I got up, wiped myself dry with a towel, changed into a new T-shirt, got back in bed, attempted to cover myself with a dry section of the sheet, and tried to sleep again. No luck. I finally got up at 3:30 a.m. and went to my office to read more emails.

An hour later, I felt exhausted and went back to bed. I next awoke at 7:30 a.m., drenched again. I removed and threw down my T-shirt in disgust. I put on my third T-shirt of the night, walked into the kitchen, and started to work on the morning's meal by polishing off a strawberry whip yogurt that checked in at 140 calories. I was around eight pounds below my usual weight and determined not to lose any more muscle. But hey, it didn't feel like such hard work anymore. Every one of those calories went down without a problem. A couple of hours later, I ate a bowl of Special K cereal, again without a hitch. I still faced each swallow with mild trepidation and felt relief as the food slid down.

Later that morning, two days after I'd come home, Rachel drove me to Dr. Drury's office in the tower adjacent to the hospital for follow-up labs. My white cell count remained above normal but had declined a little more, a somewhat reassuring result. As the process that caused the elevation resolves, the white count slowly goes down, eventually back to normal. If the cause is not resolved, then the white count will stay up or rise.

For dinner that evening, Rachel prepared chicken paprikash with Hungarian-style dumplings *(nokedli)*. I eyed my plate with trepidation, cut off a tiny piece of meat, chewed it thoroughly and swallowed apprehensively. To my relief, the food went down without a hitch. During the rest of the meal, I felt some hesitation as a morsel or two momentarily stuck in the back of my throat before sliding down. But I never once gagged, and my ability to swallow appeared to be coming back to normal on post-op day 15.

The next evening, on my fourth day home, it got there. I polished off my entire dinner with confidence, and for the first time since surgery, my swallowing felt completely normal, consistent with Marty Hopp's prediction that the problem would go away in less than one month.

What a relief! Nothing like a temporary disability to appreciate the ordinary. Swallowing with ease—pure joy. Even pills went down without a hitch. I gobbled down two and three tablets at a time, mostly to test myself, feeling more relieved than smug. Each step of progress on the road of healing provided encouragement, and this one generated unadulterated delight.

In the ensuing days, friends brought over homemade pomegranate bread, strawberries purchased at a farmers' market, and a mango cake. Because I was no longer restricted to eating mush, my appetite improved, and I slowly began regaining weight.

On post-op day 16, I went to the gym in my building and took a cautious walk on the treadmill. Amy, the physician assistant working on Dr. Trento's team, had admonished me not to do anything that could stress my sternum. The bone takes three months to heal completely. Until then, if pulled in opposite directions, the two halves could separate slightly and then fail to heal properly. That meant no lifting free weights or holding on to the elliptical's movable handles.

On subsequent days, I increased the intensity of my treadmill workouts, backing off whenever my incision began to ache. I started at three miles per hour and slowly advanced the rate up to four. Before my illness, I had routinely run on that machine at six to seven miles per hour.

I also continued making my twice-daily treks around the complex. When Rachel was out running errands or at work, I strolled alone. However, we walked together at least once every day. Sometimes I struggled to keep up with her and even asked her to slow down. My pace clearly remained much slower than my pre-surgery normal.

My chest continued to feel numb from the central incision to just outside both of my nipples. I could sense the light cotton of a T-shirt or the touch of Rachel's fingers, but their contact with my skin felt dull and strange.

I gained a greater appreciation for different levels of softness in my clothing. Some of my shirts, perfectly comfortable in the past, now felt too rough and irritated the skin over my chest. I banished the offending items from my wardrobe. Inadvertent pressure on any part of

my chest triggered a momentary spasm of pain. Whenever anyone moved in to hug me, I responded with a
defensive maneuver—holding that person off with my
palm or turning at an angle. I also explained each time
why I needed to avoid direct contact to my chest. This
soon after surgery, I didn't have to exercise such precaution often. Feeling too insecure about my energy level to
socialize, I stayed home most of the time and discouraged
visitors.

None of this was unusual or unexpected. Getting
home may have given me more familiar surroundings,
but my post-surgical body was not the same. In a way,
I had come home, but my old body, my old self wasn't
there. The social reluctance, too, was typical: many people
post-surgery feel uncomfortable about not being able to
be "themselves" with other people.

My night sweats persisted for several weeks. I would
wake up drenched in the middle of the night, change into
a new T-shirt and try to get warm again under a dry section of the top sheet. Each evening before going to bed, I
set out several T-shirts on the nearby dresser. By morning,
two or three of them lay soaking wet and crumpled by the
side of the bed. After a while, I changed strategy and hung
the wet T-shirts up on the dresser to dry. In the morning,
I could count how many of them lay on this makeshift
clothesline. Some nights, I woke up only once, giving
me hope that this ordeal was ebbing, but the next day, a
discouraging trio of T-shirts in different stages of wetness
once again rested atop the dresser.

Because my body's thermostat was off-kilter, keeping
myself warm presented a recurring challenge. Even in
Southern California, wintertime means colder outdoor

temperatures—mostly in the 50s, with lows in the upper 40s early in the morning and afternoon highs in the 60s. My hands, feet, nose, and ears frequently felt icy cold. My teeth chattered outdoors, not always but often enough to be a nuisance. Rachel generously warmed my extremities with her body heat, holding my hands against her, and massaging my feet several times daily. My usual attire at home included a pair of navy-blue sweatpants and a matching sweatshirt. Even indoors, I often wore gloves, a knit ski hat and one of Rachel's gray shawls around my neck. The shawl also brought back good memories; Rachel had purchased it during our Italy trip.

A friend joined me for a stroll around Park Place one afternoon. Having just played soccer, he wore shorts and a T-shirt while I remained bundled in my usual sweatpants, sweatshirt, warm jacket, neck shawl, ski cap, and gloves. We presented a curious contrast, walking side by side with one of us dressed for the ski slopes and the other for a stroll on the beach.

In some ways, the body's reaction to major surgery mimics aging. I remember my grandfather, when he was in his eighties and I in my teens, putting on several pairs of socks in the winter. Circulatory deficiency may have contributed to his cold feet, but he seemed to wear too many layers on the rest of his body as well. Now, at a much younger age, I was dressing like my grandfather. Not exactly, though: I didn't wear tight suspenders—and I had high hopes that this, too, would pass.

Recuperation from surgery proceeds step by step. Patients slowly resume usual activities—getting together with friends, going out to a ball game, movie, or restaurant. Initially they feel some trepidation, tire faster than before, and leave gatherings early. But slowly, as strength and endurance increase, so does confidence.

In the days following my surgery, I had no libido at all. My body had retreated into survival mode, with all my energy focused on recovery. Rachel and I cuddled, hugging each other for extended periods of time, but I sought to avoid any movement that might induce pain from my chest incision. I sensed she was afraid that our sex life might never be the same. Then, rather unexpectedly, on post-op day 23 while we were cuddling in bed as we had been the day before and the day before that, my body started to respond with desire. We cautiously approached each other and restricted our lovemaking to touching. A couple of days later, we carefully advanced to intercourse, choreographing positions and movements to spare my chest any tension or pressure. After that, as my body healed, we slowly upped the frequency and vigor of our sexual activity.

As my energy level improved, we also started going out more often. We visited the nearby Mormon Temple to admire the colorful display of lights throughout their garden and attend a bell concert performance in their visitors' center. We drove to the Grove, an open-air shopping mall, to see its tall, lavishly decorated Christmas tree and artful department store displays. Being part of the holidays and cultural events helped me feel that I was rejoining humanity.

By mid-December, my energy level was strong enough to stay up all day without taking rest periods in bed. I still needed to be careful to avoid pain caused by any inadvertent movement that put a strain on my chest—but I could feel the progress.

Being fit may not have prevented me from coming down with heart disease, but it helped me recuperate. Although I had been disappointed by my brief physical therapy session at the hospital, the therapist was right—I was able to get around my home without assistance. People who start out less fit may not be so fortunate. A major illness causes frailty. If this new frailty is added to preexisting frailty, it may necessitate recuperation in a rehab unit for a while. After going home, some people may require a full-time caretaker or equipment such as a walker or a shower chair. Some may even need to have rails or a stair elevator installed in their homes. Of course, everyone needs help after a major illness. I was fortunate to have Rachel's capable and loving assistance throughout my recuperation.

Chapter 13

Rehabbing: The Power
of the Mind and Body

It is much more important to know what sort
of a patient has a disease than what sort of a
disease a patient has.

—Dr. William Osler, cofounder of the
Johns Hopkins University School of Medicine

D r. Drury and the cardiac surgery team had advised me
to enroll in a supervised exercise program six weeks
after my surgery. On post-op day 42, I registered at the
Cedars-Sinai Preventive and Rehabilitative Cardiac Center, a few blocks away from the main hospital.

The process began with filling out a lengthy ques-
tionnaire in the waiting lounge. While I wrote down my
answers, already-enrolled clients, looking frail and over
70, shuffled through on their way to the rehab gym.
Some pushed walkers; others used canes. One woman
stopped to chat with Rachel. "This is a wonderful place,"
she gushed. "I've been coming here for years."

For years? That didn't sound encouraging. My goal for
rehab was to get back to my previous normal as quickly
as possible.

After a visit with the medical director of the unit, I
went to the rehab gym and Rachel left to run errands. A

young nurse took my baseline blood pressure and counted my resting pulse rate. Then, given a choice of upright and reclining stationary bikes, treadmills, and stair climbers, I elected to start on a treadmill. The nurse set its rate at 2.5 miles per hour with no incline. That felt too slow to me, so I raised the speed to 3 miles per hour. She came by to check on me and reduced the pace down to 2.8 miles per hour, warning me that strenuous exercise too soon can be dangerous.

"You can advance to three miles per hour next time. It'll be safer that way."

She recorded my blood pressure and pulse again and noted that they remained in a healthy range. After ten minutes of leisurely walking, my session on the treadmill was over and I moved to a reclining bike. Ten minutes of light pedaling later, with my time up, the nurse again checked my vital signs and told me, "You did very well for your first session."

"I think I can do a lot more than this," I replied. "I've been exercising more vigorously on my own at home."

"Don't worry. Wait till next time. We'll get you doing plenty more progressively."

The following day in rehab, things were much the same. I was disappointed and frustrated. Of course I didn't want to push myself to a level of exertion that would harm my health, but the pace of my workout at rehab amounted to no more than a stroll. At this rate, getting back to my normal exercise level would indeed take years.

The purpose of cardiac rehab is to increase exercise capability safely over time. While patients exercise, their blood pressure and heart rate are checked at frequent intervals. Medical intervention is readily available for those who develop chest pain or any other sign of distress.

Although the staff let me advance the intensity of my workouts at succeeding sessions, they did so very slowly. They appeared to follow a preordained schedule and would not budge from it despite my desire to advance more rapidly.

After my eighth visit to rehab, on December 30, I felt confident I could manage my exercise regimen just as safely and more effectively at home. I knew enough not to push myself to the point of pain or exhaustion, but I didn't want to be limited to exercise that didn't even feel like exercise. Besides, I could measure my blood pressure and count my pulse rate as accurately as the nurses at rehab. I felt the staff was holding me back, slowing down my progress. So, I switched to a physician-monitored exercise program—with me as the monitoring physician.

Being a doctor gave me the confidence that I could manage my workouts safely. However, the tools to design a healthy exercise program are not exclusive to medical personnel. Blood pressure measuring systems intended for self-use are sold in drugstores, and a watch with a second hand or phone with a stopwatch make checking pulse rates a cinch. An irregular pulse can be felt with a finger, and smartwatches can diagnose atrial fibrillation. With a bit of self-education, careful individuals can adequately monitor their own exercise programs. Of course, the more you know to begin with, the easier this is. Being a doctor was an advantage.

For several weeks, every time we went somewhere by car, Rachel drove. I sat with the pillow from the hospital in front of me, shielding my chest from the pressure of the seatbelt. I even pushed the seatbelt away from the pillow to keep it from hurting the tender skin over my sternum.

Some of my appointments had to be scheduled for days when Rachel needed to attend to her real estate deals, so I had to start driving. On post-op day 43, I got behind the wheel for the first time since my surgery. The height of the pillow, which came up past my chin, presented the most immediate problem. Rachel cut the padding in half and sewed the edges together to produce a more compact model. The pressure from the seatbelt, even cushioned by the custom-made pillow, continued to hurt enough to bother me after only a few minutes. While waiting at stoplights, I pushed the chest strap out to relieve the pain. Searching for a way to eliminate my discomfort, I tucked the chest strap below my left arm, converting it into a second lap belt. That may not conform to recommended safety rules, but under the circumstances, I felt I could probably talk my way out of a ticket if stopped. Despite the annoying inconveniences that came with driving, the freedom to get around on my own provided another encouraging sign of my step-by-step progress toward normalcy.

Recuperating from an illness calls for adaptations. It might require making changes in a rehab exercise program that's progressing too slowly. Customization, such as Rachel cutting a pillow down to size, can also help.

Some innovations may be questionable and limited to a brief time, like neutralizing a chest strap while driving. It may take a pillow, a cane, or a warm pack to ease aches that hold a patient back. A little MacGyvering can go a long way to eliminate obstacles on the road to recovery.

People with disabilities, temporary and permanent, have designed their own innovations, alone or with the help of engineers and technicians. Customized cars allow a person missing an arm or two to drive around town. A woman who became blind memorized the steps it took to get from one part of her apartment to another. If you didn't know she was blind, you wouldn't have detected it from the way she opened doors and walked around furniture. She also used a variety of devices that helped her become self-sufficient. A simple sensor attached to the side of a coffee cup beeped when fluid reached it, and made it easy for her to fill the mug without spilling a drop. Every time I visited her, I was impressed by her ability to cope and thrive.

Chapter 14

Reflections:
A Shift in Perspectives

When a man knows he is to be hanged in a fortnight, it concentrates his mind wonderfully.

—Samuel Johnson

H eart surgery doesn't quite rise to the level of a hanging. More like a Taser shock, it stuns the body and mind with enough jolt to generate extensive self-reflection.

A life-endangering event followed by lots of free time tends to inspire contemplation about fundamental issues. While recuperating from my surgery, I had opportunity to reflect on life in general and on mine in particular.

Throughout my illness, I had (mostly) maintained a positive outlook. I never doubted I would survive, but at times feared being limited in my ability to live as well as before. *Will I be able to be as active? Will I be as competent?* My goal was to be able to answer both those questions in the affirmative. I wanted my previous life back, to be my former self again, both physically and mentally.

Almost all surgery patients share these fears or others such as: *Will I be a burden? Will the pain last forever? Will I be able to cope financially?*

An estimated 30 to 40 percent of CABG patients suffer some level of depression around the time of their surgery.

The incidence of depression for patients hospitalized for other reasons may be similar. That increases morbidity, both because of biochemical changes associated with depression and because of patients' diminished ability to work on their rehabilitation.

Viktor Frankl, a psychiatrist and concentration camp survivor, observed that even in places as hellish as those prisons, "the last of human freedoms," the one that remains after a person is deprived of all else, is "the ability to choose one's attitude in a given set of circumstances." Even in far less awful situations, exercising that freedom by choosing a positive attitude can make a significant difference. It sounds so simple, but of course, it's easier said than done.

My predisposition to focus on the positive served me well during my recuperation. Every few days, I took an inventory of the progress I had made since surgery. That piggybacked on a habit that I had started in my teens. On my birthdays and every New Year's Day, I reflected on the prior months to select recent positive events that made me feel fortunate and grateful. Only as an adult, and perhaps only after seeing the despair of patients with depression, did I realize how lucky I had been all along to possess this tendency, another reason to feel fortunate.

A major illness changes a person's equilibrium. Some people who sink into depression following CABG may also have had an optimistic nature. Like coronary artery disease, depression can sneak up even on someone who does everything right. Fortunately, it didn't on me.

During my reflections, I went through an inventory, evaluating my life prior and subsequent to my surgery. I was grateful that my physiological requirements of food, water, and shelter were secure. Until my current health crisis, I had been confident of my safety, but heart disease had introduced an unwelcome element of insecurity that I wanted and needed to reduce.

Maintaining good health after heart surgery called for a new knowledge-based plan of exercise, diet, and medication. I hoped my doctors and I would come up with a regimen that would succeed for a long time. However, I felt some trepidation about this: I felt that healthwise, I had done most things right in the past, yet still wound up needing open-heart surgery.

Viktor Frankl observed that "man is not destroyed by suffering; he is destroyed by suffering without meaning." I wanted to learn something from this experience. Surgery and hospitalization create many losses—of time, sense of self, the narratives of our lives; a good recovery is not only about restoration, it is also about creating something new, a positive change.

Spirituality can give meaning to suffering, help people find hope. Prayer and meditation have a soothing effect, promote relaxation, and reduce stress. Belonging to a religious community helps many people recover from suffering, including the distress caused by a health crisis. Faith can provide a sense of purpose and meaning to life. A religious community also provides social support. Members of a congregation may help out with gifts of food, run errands, and give comfort. All these factors combine to enhance healing.

Those of us not actively involved in religious observance need to find similar solace and inspiration from other sources. My motivation came from an intense desire to reclaim the life I had lived. My social support came from family and friends. During my recovery, I also committed to write about my experience to help others live through similar health crises. The idea that something positive could come out of my travails added to my resolve to recover quickly and fully.

Robert F. Kennedy said, "The purpose of life is to contribute in some way to making things better." Martin Luther King Jr. declared, "Life's most persistent and urgent question is, 'What are you doing for others?'" According to their tradition, Jews are called to participate in *tikkun olam*, which translates as "improving the world."

Given a new lease on life, people have a tendency to focus on making it more meaningful. As I recuperated, I felt an obligation to remember that.

I also wanted to take the time to show gratitude for my good fortune. Though at the time I didn't think about how showing gratitude might benefit me, it is known to confer a host of benefits to the grateful, from better mental health, sleep, and resiliency to lower levels of anxiety and depression and a greater sense of overall well-being. Showing gratitude, focusing on what we have to be grateful for, is a powerful way to foster a positive mindset.[1]

To recognize exemplary care, Cedars acknowledges hospital staff commended by patients through a program called "Standing Ovation." I felt that virtually all my doctors, nurses, therapists, and technicians deserved Standing Ovations. I left the hospital with a handful of forms and filled them out during my first week home. I wrote one for Inna, noting her kindness in helping me bathe and consequently feel so much better upon my arrival on 6 Northeast. I sent Standing Ovations to several of the RNs who had paid attention to my comfort as well as my safety. I regretted that I couldn't remember the names of some very deserving nurses who took care of me shortly after surgery, at a time when I was less alert. And of course, I wanted to give extra-special recognition to Marietta, the speech therapist whose expertise proved crucial to diagnosing my swallowing problem.

During the December holiday season, I combined my visits to doctors' offices with delivering gifts of champagne and other goodies to several of my doctors, nurses, and therapists. I did this to further express my appreciation for their capable and kind care. Perhaps I also wanted to be a memorable patient, but for a good reason.

PART IV

RECOVERY TO RENEWAL

Chapter 15

The Long and Short of Dying: Contemplating Mortality

> The meaning of life is that it stops.
>
> —Franz Kafka

Cardiac illness is sudden death incarnate. It therefore tends to inspire thoughts about mortality. Although I didn't think my death was imminent at any point before or after my surgery, the possibility lurked in the background like a haunting, recurring melody in the soundtrack of a movie.

Kafka's assessment in the epigraph above sounds too gloomy to me. Our actions have consequences beyond our years and give lasting meaning to our lives. Death gives urgency to life and looms as the final deadline to all we can accomplish, but it doesn't define life. What we do during our lives, our positive and negative effects on others, has its own consequential meaning. We can strive to help improve the lives of others.

No matter how you look at dying, the final moment of earthly life arrives in one of two ways. Death can result from an illness that develops in a roughly predictable manner, occurring within an expected time range. Patients with terminal cancer can take such a downhill course. Conversely, death can arrive without warning, within minutes, from an event like a sudden cardiac arrest or a car crash.

At 94, my father looked and acted like a man 20 years younger. To avoid any problems with the vision test for renewing his driver's license, he had cataract surgery. A week later, on an October morning, Dad trimmed the bushes in his garden and tended to the birds-of-paradise that had begun to bloom in front of the house. He then took his customary mile-long walk around the neighborhood, observing elm, maple, and palm trees and the squirrels that scampered around them.

That afternoon, feeling weak and lightheaded, Dad checked his blood pressure and noted that it was below normal. For the next several hours, his blood pressure cycled up and down 10 to 25 points while his energy level waxed and waned. In the evening, he called me to discuss whether he should go to the hospital. Since he was then feeling better, we decided to wait and see how the next hours went. Around 9:00 p.m., after a recurrence of his symptoms, I drove Dad to Cedars-Sinai Medical Center.

As we waited for the emergency room doctor, my father began feeling better. "Perhaps coming here wasn't necessary. I feel okay now," he said.

When the ER doctor arrived, Dad gave him a detailed description of the day's events, complete with hourly blood pressures and pulse rates. The physician looked down at the chart, then back at my father. "How can I be like you when I'm 94?" he asked. "Heck, how can I be like you now? I don't often get such a good history from people of any age."

My father's ECG looked unchanged; his vital signs and labs measured within normal limits. He sat upright briskly when the doctor asked to listen to his lungs. Still, given my father's earlier low blood pressure and his age, the ER doc recommended overnight hospital observation.

After my father was settled in his room, I prepared to go home to get some sleep since I had cases scheduled for early in the morning. As I approached the door of his hospital room, my father said, "Wait. Don't go. I don't feel good."

His head rolled back. I rushed to his bedside.

"Dad, are you okay?"

No response. I shook him, then shook him again more vigorously. Still no response. I pushed the code blue button on the wall behind the bed and felt for a carotid artery pulse. Nothing. The code team arrived to perform CPR.

The code leader, a senior resident, directed six others. The intern pumped on Dad's chest; a resident started a large-bore IV; one nurse opened the drug cart, ready to draw up resuscitative meds; another recorded all the meds given; a respiratory tech took up her position by the head of the bed and administered oxygen with a mask. A resident and a medical student connected pads for recording rhythm and delivering electric shocks. A heart with no electrical activity can't be revived. The monitor showed a shockable rhythm. Everyone stepped away from the bed. A jolt rocked my father's body.

When a life-sustaining heart rhythm didn't promptly return, the code leader called for intubation. I was the only anesthesiologist in the room, by far the most experienced at performing that maneuver. I opened my father's mouth and inserted the breathing tube into his trachea.

For a procedure that can bridge the abyss between life and death, the steps of cardiopulmonary resuscitation are cookbook simple. Compress chest, ventilate lungs, apply electric shocks, inject resuscitative drugs. Meanwhile the team analyzes the reasons for the cardiac arrest, searching for a treatable cause. The sequence can be repeated, giving additional medicines before each shock, but the chances of survival diminish over time. If the heart doesn't respond adequately after several shocks, continuing the effort becomes futile. At that point, the physician in charge "calls the code," halting further treatment and declaring the patient deceased.

After several cycles of resuscitation with no response, the effort to restart my father's heart appeared to be failing. I clung to the wall behind the bed, stunned. As this patient's son, I wanted the resuscitation to continue. Dad was a retired electronics engineer, a brilliant and kind man. He enjoyed lively discussions, knew how to repair electrical appliances, loved hiking, and travel. When Dad was 86, we trekked in the Canadian Rockies together. Having attended numerous code blues, I stood there, looking on, feeling both the past with my father and our future slipping away.

"How old is this patient?" the code leader asked.

"94," someone replied.

The code leader hesitated.

If anyone in the room knew the patient was my father, I was not aware of it. I could have been a random anesthesiologist who happened to be nearby when the patient arrested. Of course, my relationship should have made no difference.

"He's completely with it and active," I interjected. "Very healthy, like a man much younger."

The team members all looked at me. "He hasn't responded to six shocks," said the code leader, eyeing me dubiously.

Before he could say, "I'm calling this code," the words, "He's my father," blurted out of me.

A silence followed. The resuscitation continued.

The next shock likewise produced no viable rhythm. By then, the prospects of my father leaving the hospital without hypoxic brain damage after CPR for that long were approaching nil. Years earlier, Dad had signed a living will, specifying that he didn't want life-prolonging measures in such a situation.

My father's internist had been called and wanted to talk with me. Knowing the inevitable, I reluctantly stepped out of the room and picked up the phone at the nursing station. Minutes later, while I was still on the phone, the code team filed out. They didn't have to tell me the outcome. As they shuffled by, the code leader paused to express sympathy. He told me I could go back into the room and be with my father until transporters from the morgue arrived.

In the now silent room my father looked calm, his eyes closed as if asleep. Someone, probably the respiratory tech, had removed the breathing tube and closed his mouth. I sat on the edge of the bed and clutched his right hand. Though lifeless, it was still warm.

Two men dressed all in white arrived. I stood back as they covered my father's face with a white sheet, lifted his body onto a rolling gurney, and covered him with a metal shield. They rolled the gurney out of the room. I watched it recede down the hallway. Nurses and doctors stepped out of the way. They knew what such a metal shield atop a gurney meant.

The death of a patient sometimes feels inevitable, sometimes like a defeat, often both. In this case, we had done everything that we knew how to do. It was enough but not good enough. As I watched my father being rolled away, I felt the crushing weight of forever losing an irre-placeable part of my life.

It was 5:00 a.m. The morning shift of doctors and nurses arrived. The ordinariness of the scene felt jarringly surreal. I phoned the operating room scheduling nurse to tell her someone else would have to cover my cases, then headed to my father's home.

The Spanish-style house I grew up in felt cold and empty. I slowly wandered from room to lonely room. My father's yellow armchair, the one he sat in while reading *TIME* and watching the evening news, looked forlorn and useless. So did the cream-colored chair nearby, the one I sat in while we discussed current events, history, upcom-ing trips. In my father's bedroom, the bed was neatly made. My childhood room still held the same single bed, small desk, and diplomas from high school, college, and medical school my mother had framed. It dawned on me that the place now felt like a museum filled with artifacts from the past. I was the last surviving member of my birth family, the lone possessor of the memory of the life once lived in this house.

By contrast, my mother's death at age 77 from pancreatic cancer was slow. Two years earlier, she and my father had celebrated their fiftieth wedding anniversary. That December, Mom was diagnosed with a metastatic tumor. In situations like hers, her oncologist told her, the progression of the illness typically results in death within six months. Chemotherapy could prolong her life but also make her sick. If there were events she wanted to live to see six months from then, chemotherapy might be worthwhile. If quality time was the objective, taking toxic compounds that—while stretching the calendar—would cause pain, nausea, diarrhea, and other nasty symptoms made little sense.

Mom declined chemotherapy. She died four months later. Still, in the interlude preceding her death, she had the chance to say goodbye to family and friends, providing all of us some comfort amid the inevitable sadness. We had time to express love and gratitude for what we had contributed to each other's lives. Mom made an effort to teach Dad a few cooking skills, so he could better take care of his nutrition after her passing. Before getting too weak, she took him grocery shopping and provided pointers while he placed simple meals in the oven. Mom told Dad that he was the great love of her life and knew that she was his. She also said that he had her blessing to find another lady for companionship and love after her passing, since she believed he would be happier that way. Dad also expressed his love for Mom, and found a measure of comfort in that opportunity.

With most everything clearly stated, Mom passed her final days calmly, courageously, and stoically. Near the end, pain medication made her sleepy even during daytime. She slipped into unconsciousness in the middle of an April night, never to wake again.

Lots of people claim some variation of "The doctors gave her six months to live, but she stayed alive for five years." Or conversely, "She died in less than six weeks." This is a misunderstanding of what doctors actually say, or even have the know-how to say. They can't predict an event weeks, months, or years away with clockwork accuracy. Physicians can tell you the average time people live with a particular diagnosis. They can't foretell how an individual patient with an illness such as pancreatic cancer will respond to treatment. They don't have the divine ability to predict the exact course of every patient's illness.

In my father's house that day, I found a notebook he'd prepared with instructions on what I needed to do when he passed—inform friends and relatives, pay bills, stop subscriptions. I wandered back into the living room, sat in the cream-colored armchair, and stared at the empty yellow one. Several minutes went by, maybe longer. The phone rang, jolting me out of my stupor. The next-door neighbor called to remind my father to turn off the porch night-light. When I told her that he had passed away, she argued, "No! He couldn't have. I saw him yesterday. He was trimming the hedges. We talked. He was fine."

Over the next several days, friends and family expressed similar disbelief. Dad had planned to see a movie later that week with a lady friend.

Even though my father lived to an age 17 years older than my mother, his passing caught people by surprise. However, he escaped feeling sick and enduring progressive deterioration of the ability to live life as he wanted. His family didn't have to witness his slow decline. But we didn't have a chance for final goodbyes.

Of the two ways of dying, most people express a preference—for themselves—for abrupt surprise. Many have told me my father was lucky to have lived a long life and then died suddenly, with minimal suffering. The downside is the lack of opportunity for final expressions of affection and gratitude. Family and close friends feel a void, not just from losing the deceased but from the loss of the opportunity to say goodbye.

With my mother, we started mourning before she passed away. When that day arrived, we were more prepared. Perhaps my father's passing shouldn't have been totally unexpected at his age. But with no imminent signals beforehand, it caught us all off guard. The sudden blow hit harder than the anticipated one. Reaching the milestone of acceptance took longer, maybe even longer than the combined duration of mourning before and after my mother died.

Of course, mourning never really ends. We just move on. I continue to miss both my parents and am comforted by memories of them.

My mother and father both died at a relatively advanced age. Would a longer warning help ease the passing of someone younger?

Neurosurgeon Paul Kalanithi was 36 and completing his final year of residency at Stanford when he was diagnosed with stage IV lung cancer. Though devastated, Kalanithi still had the opportunity to decide how to spend the rest of his life. In the 22 months between his diagnosis and death, he finished his residency, fathered a daughter, and wrote an amazing book *(When Breath Becomes Air)*. The warning gave Kalanithi the chance to use his remaining days to produce an enduring positive impact. It also gave his wife and others dear to him the opportunity to express their love. If Kalanithi had died suddenly, he would not have written his book, not have had a child, and had fewer heartfelt discussions with loved ones. If anything, a warning may be even more helpful to everyone involved when death arrives at a younger age.

Death of a loved one inevitably brings sadness. Watching that person's quality of life deteriorate over time is painful. But having an opportunity to express gratitude for what that mother, father, child, or friend has meant to you can help lessen the ache. A sudden death eliminates the slow decline, but also the opportunity for a proper goodbye. Each way of dying has its advantages and its downsides.

My cardiac condition could have resulted in an abrupt death, much like my father's, but it would have occurred when I was 32 years younger than the age at which he died. That made me too young to be considered lucky to die suddenly but too old to have died young. Death at an awkward in-between age? No, thanks. Having escaped that fate with the help of modern medicine, I neither know how my end will come, nor which way I would prefer. Prior to my illness, I had been aware of the two possibilities but had never given the slightest thought about them for myself. Heart surgery inspired me, or perhaps forced me, to reflect on the past, present, future, and the fundamental issues of life and death. It didn't hand me any easy answers.

Chapter 16

Edging to Normal:
The Precipice of Healthy

Some people see the glass half full. Others see it half empty. I see a glass that's twice as big as it needs to be.

—George Carlin

As recuperation continues, patients arrive at a point when they're not yet healthy enough to work but healthy enough to do a lot. This time period starts to resemble a vacation—but not quite, due to lingering symptoms. The extra leisure time frees up patients to engage in activities that lift their spirits, things they had previously wished to do but work got in the way.

This, too, is an important part of recovery. Creating something new requires some distance, some space.

For me, although my chest remained exquisitely tender, my energy level continued to steadily improve, and was approaching close to normal.

Since starting work after my residency, for more than thirty years ago, I had taken the opportunity to travel during each of my vacations, always eager to explore a new part of the world. Now I enjoyed the pleasure of leisure time at home.

I had more opportunities to survey Christmas decorations around town, imbibe the festive atmosphere of the season, stroll on Santa Monica Beach with Rachel, and take classes on MacBook and iPhoto at the local Apple store. Who knew that coming down with heart disease was a path to computer education?

In the days immediately after my operation, my voice sounded weak and raspy. Perhaps the breathing tube had traumatized my vocal cords during intubation. The trauma of surgery might have caused inflammation to the area around the vocal cords or the nerves that control it. My general weakness likely contributed to the vocal frailty as well. After major surgery, there are often additional problems like this that remind us that our body has been through a lot, that recovery is ongoing.

My voice slowly regained most of its strength, but it remained weaker than usual throughout much of my recuperation. I went for a speech therapy evaluation near the end of December and then to three therapy sessions in January. Every day between visits, I practiced vocal exercises prescribed by the speech therapist. By the end of January, my voice sounded normal.

Eventually the twelfth week after my surgery arrived, the last week before my scheduled return to work. I certainly felt strong enough to perform my job but had mixed emotions. I enjoyed the freedom to do whatever whenever with no responsibility to show up anywhere on schedule, but I knew it was time to get back to real life.

On the Sunday before my return to work, I took a long walk in my neighborhood, worked out on the elliptical machine in my building, and lifted light weights. I went to bed at 9:30 p.m. and set the alarm on my clock radio for the first time in three months.

My illness-generated semi-vacation ended on post-op day 88, Monday, January 31. After three months away from work, I drove to the hospital a bit apprehensive about diving back into the busy schedule and responsibilities of my job.

Over 100 anesthesiologists worked at Cedars-Sinai, in operating rooms on five different floors of the main hospital building and in a variety of other areas, including a cystoscopy suite, a gastrointestinal endoscopy lab, the cardiac cath lab, interventional radiology, and several outpatient surgicenters. For that first day, I had arranged to do cases in one of my favorite areas in the hospital. As soon as I walked through the door of that suite, several of the nurses and aides greeted me with bright smiles and open arms.

"Welcome back."

"Great to see you," they said, one after the other. We hugged, but I took care to keep everyone away from my still tender chest, telling everybody why and turning slightly to make contact with only my side.

Above my anesthesia machine, I saw a red banner stretching across the back wall with large black block letters: "Welcome Home." I had anticipated a warm welcome; their wholehearted effort went beyond my expectations. When I walked to our snack area, I received a gift package of chips and other goodies, each item labeled "heart healthy."

I quickly felt at home in the haven of my work family. I also felt comfortable back on the job. I only needed extra help with one task. At the conclusion of a procedure, we sometimes elevate the patient's torso and head to make breathing easier. Whenever that was appropriate, I asked a nurse or another doctor to lift the upper part of the gurney, since doing so myself would have put tension on my chest.

After the conclusion of my lineup, I walked over to the Anesthesiology Department office. Before I got there, I ran into one of the vascular surgeons in the hallway. "Hey, good to see you back, Andy," he said, with a big smile. I got the same greeting from our secretaries and felt that it was indeed good to be back where I belonged, in my familiar role at my home away from home.

The rest of the week whisked by smoothly. The following Monday morning, feeling totally relaxed while driving to the hospital I noted, "What a difference a week makes." Just like riding a bike after a long hiatus, taking care of patients again felt as natural as if I had never taken a break. That's what I had expected, but it was reassuring to see it come to pass. I was back—not yet 100 percent my normal self, but getting close.

Sixteen weeks after my surgery, on post-op day 112, February 24, I went for a follow-up visit with Dr. Drury. Everything checked out: ECG unchanged, slight residual anemia but approaching a normal red blood cell count, white blood cell count normal, no sign of any problems.

"At this point, there are no limitations on your activities. You can do anything . . . except maybe bench press 200 pounds," Kevin told me.

"So bungee jumping is okay?" I asked.

"No. That's out, too."

Somewhere around this time, my chest tenderness diminished to the point that the shoulder straps of seatbelts no longer bothered me. The area of numbness gradually narrowed to an inch on either side of the scar over my sternum. Rachel pointed out that my chest looked a lot like a happy face cartoon, with my nipples representing the eyes, the central incision the nose and the scars from the four drain sites outlining the mouth, slightly upturned on my right side to form a wry smile. I began telling people that the only remaining visible evidence of my surgery was a happy face.

By this time, my life had returned to normal. I was working full-time, exercising regularly, writing, and going to movies, plays, concerts, and sporting events.

One of my colleagues remarked that he and his wife saw me bounding across the plaza level of the hospital one morning. "Isn't that Andy Kadar? Didn't he have heart surgery a little while ago?" she asked. "Sure doesn't look sick anymore."

Several weeks after my return to the OR, I was work-ing on the sixth floor, pushing a patient on a gurney through the same back corridor that I had been rolled down a few months earlier. Now, however, I was back in my appropriate role, injecting a sedative through the patient's IV. This time, nobody remarked about me being on the wrong side of the bed. The stars and planets in the universe had returned to their rightful places. I felt fit and all was well. Triumphant music played silently in my head as we marched toward the OR.

Twelve months after my surgery, I returned to Dr. Drury's office for a follow-up exercise tolerance test, also known as a stress test. It took place in the same cluttered room as the year before, but this time I strode in feeling confident and healthy.

An exercise tolerance test begins with a technician placing conducting leads on the subject and connecting these to a 12-lead ECG. Then the patient steps onto a treadmill. Initially the operator sets the treadmill to a slow speed, allowing the patient to warm up and the exam-iner to detect problems with minimal exercise. During my exam the prior year, Kevin started me at the prescribed speed of 1.7 miles per hour and a 10-degree incline. After 2 minutes and 40 seconds, I had felt burning in my chest and showed clear signs of *ischemia* (inadequate blood supply) on multiple ECG leads, prompting Kevin to halt the test. If I had remained symptom-free and showed no abnormalities on the ECG, we would have proceeded after three minutes to the next stage of testing by increasing the speed and raising the angle of the treadmill until I complained of exhaustion or showed signs or symptoms of ischemia. If that didn't happen, the test would have continued until my heart rate reached at least 85 percent but not more than 100 percent of my estimated maximum heart rate. The formula for calculating that number is 220 minus your age. On the anniversary of my surgery, for me, that came to 157.

This time, I blew past 2 minutes and 40 seconds without breaking a sweat or feeling the slightest distress. We advanced to the next stage and then to additional higher stages. As the speed and incline rose, my heart rate started going up. During stage five, with the treadmill humming along at five miles per hour on an 18-degree incline, my heart speed reached 133.

"You can stop now if you want," Kevin told me. "You've reached eighty-five percent of your maximum heart rate."

"Nah, I feel fine. Let's continue."

Two minutes and 40 seconds into stage five, my heart rate reached 157 and Kevin turned the treadmill off.

"Hey, I feel fine. I can keep going."

Kevin assured me that there was nothing to be gained by going past my calculated maximum heart rate.

"But I was only twenty seconds . . ."

He didn't let me finish. "Be happy you got as far as you did. Be happy that you're doing so well."

"I am, Kevin . . . I most certainly am."

Kevin had gradually reduced the number of medicines he prescribed for me from the original 16 pills daily on discharge from the hospital. The antibiotic dropped out first, no longer necessary after my incisions healed. The arrhythmia medicine amiodarone went next, not needed after over a month of normal heart rhythm. Initially I took two medicines to reduce stomach acidity and thereby prevent heartburn and ulcers. Kevin cut that down to one and eventually to only as needed.

I initially took two medicines that improve the chances of survival after cardiac surgery, an ACE (angiotensin-converting enzyme) inhibitor (lisinopril) and a beta blocker (metoprolol). ACE inhibitors lower blood pressure and allow the heart to do its job with less effort. Metoprolol relaxes the arteries and decreases heart rate. Both those actions reduce the amount of work the heart needs to perform.

An adage in medicine states that anything powerful enough to do a lot of good is powerful enough to do a lot of harm. Both ACE inhibitors and beta blockers carry a long and frightful list of potential side effects, some life-threatening and others just annoying. Lisinopril often causes coughing and less frequently causes hoarseness. With my voice still weak and sometimes hoarse nine weeks after surgery, I asked Kevin about discontinuing lisinopril. He agreed it was safe by then to be on only one cardio-protective drug, the metoprolol. I still take it two years post-op, since beta blockers seem to enhance long-term survival after coronary artery bypass surgery.

I also continue to take low-dose aspirin daily and a medicine to lower my cholesterol. I had already been on a cholesterol-reducing drug before my surgery but am now on a more powerful, newer, and therefore more expensive version that lowers my blood lipids even more.

The benefits of taking any medicine have to be balanced against its side effects and potential side effects—including previously unreported and therefore unknown side effects. After a major operation, this calls for frequent changes in the number of prescriptions and their doses. Later on, fewer adjustments are necessary, but as a disease process recedes and advances, as newer more effective drugs are introduced, a patient's medicine regimen will continue to require adjustments to achieve the best possible level of health.

My current pharmaceutical regimen is simple. Of course, I would prefer not to be reliant on medicines at all, but it's a minor nuisance well worth its protective effect.

In 2010, *U.S. News and World Report* ranked Cedars-Sinai's Cardiology and Heart Surgery as the fifteenth-best among hospitals in the United States. The exact position of a medical center in such a highly subjective ranking needs to be taken with not just a grain but a whole mountain of salt. Nevertheless, inclusion on the list indicates that a hospital has a highly regarded, large, and successful department that achieves results as good as anywhere. In any given year, the mortality rate between the hospital that the magazine's editors rank as number 1 and the one they list as number 25 is likely to be negligible.

For cardiac surgery, really for any procedure, it's best to be at a hospital that does a lot of it. The staff will be familiar with what a good recovery looks like, can recognize deviations from it promptly, and intervene effectively. When I went into atrial fibrillation, my nurse noted it immediately and called an intensivist to treat it right away. At least 100 open-heart procedures per year are considered the minimum to acquire such familiarity with cardiac surgery.

Cedars-Sinai surgeons performed 829 open-heart surgeries in the year I had mine. These included valve replacements, repairs of congenital heart defects, heart transplants, and 171 CABGs. Of the CABGs, 87 were the same type as mine, first-time open-heart surgeries not combined with any other procedures like valve replacement.

Each of those 87 patients went home alive. I don't know how many of *U.S. News and World Report's* top fourteen ranked hospitals had 100 percent survival rates among comparable patients, but we can safely conclude that none of them did better. (Rankings change from year to year. In 2023, *U.S. News and World Report* rated Cedars-Sinai number 2 in the nation in heart surgery.)

For almost any illness, most Americans can find state-of-the-art high-quality care at a medical center near their home. Somebody living in a major metropolitan area like Los Angeles definitely can.

For simple and common procedures, a good community hospital can deliver care as well as an internationally renowned medical center. For a hernia repair, breast biopsy, or an appendectomy, a well-equipped and well-staffed small hospital, even one with only a few operating rooms, can produce results as good as Cedars-Sinai or the Mayo Clinic. They also have the advantage of being close and more convenient for patients who live near them. But such hospitals are usually not equipped to perform brain tumor resections or open-heart surgery. For these more complex operations, it's best to go to a medical center that performs many of them, where—and this is worth repeating—not only the doctors but also the nurses and other staff have extensive experience taking care of such patients.

Cedars-Sinai doctors, registered nurses, licensed vocational nurses, speech therapists, and other personnel took care of me with expertise and compassion. Many people have asked me if my care was so good because I'm a doctor. The answer is a definite "maybe" and calls for an explanation.

The details of my medical procedures did not deviate from the usual and customary standard of care. However, being at the hospital where I work undoubtedly made my experience easier. I had seen my doctors and nurses treat other patients capably and successfully. I never doubted I was in good hands. Having confidence in your healthcare team reduces anxiety, and I had the advantage of having full confidence in mine.

I received and much appreciated words of encouragement from colleagues who passed me in the hallway or dropped by to visit. My recuperation began in a setting both familiar and comfortable to me, practically my second home. Sick people who find themselves in a large confusing building may have a harder time adjusting simultaneously to their role as a patient and the strange surroundings.

I also took advantage of knowing the ropes and knowing other physicians on the staff a few times during my hospitalization. When frustrated by the lack of progress on my swallowing problem, I got the ball rolling a bit faster by contacting a gastroenterologist on my own. If I didn't have that opportunity, I would have had to work harder to convince my primary doctor of the level of misery my swallowing disability was causing. Most likely, the delay involved in getting to the bottom of the problem would have been anywhere from a few hours to one day.

I was able to get my hiccup medicine dose adjusted fairly quickly by knowing how to argue effectively for it. I could also make a good case for stopping the oversized potassium tablet that caused me so much distress. All these measures made my recuperation easier and made me feel better. None affected the eventual outcome.

Lay patients can also advocate for changes in their treatment by providing information and asking questions. If taking a medicine, such as my potassium, causes difficulty, letting your doctors know can lead to a beneficial substitution. Something along the lines of "This is causing me problems. Can we do something else instead?" could lead to elimination of distress. Of course, all such discussions should be conducted without hostility. Your doctors and nurses are on your side. They are dedicated to making your recuperation as easy and problem-free as possible. Smart patients do for their caregivers what the movie sports agent Jerry Maguire asked of his client, "Help me help you." Getting well is a team effort.

Throughout my recuperation, I felt reassured by knowing what symptoms require prompt medical attention. Having the ability to monitor myself allowed me to take charge of my rehab exercise program. Compared to the average patient, I had a greater ability to modify my care and thereby make my recuperation more comfortable and less stressful. The psychological impact of that surely had a significant positive effect on my mood. Prudent questioning can help lay patients modify their treatments as well and can lead to a feeling of greater influence over their situation.

I do want to point out again that every one of the 87 patients who underwent the same type of surgery as mine at the same hospital during the same year went home alive. Most actually suffered fewer complications and went home sooner. The advantages I enjoyed made my recuperation somewhat easier but produced no difference to the eventual outcome.

Doctors, nurses, therapists, technicians, dieticians, and other hospital workers devoted many hours and lots of effort to my treatment. They used expensive equipment like a heart-lung machine, ventilators, and video X-ray machines. The time and material resources involved in my care, in the care of any CABG patient, add up to a sizable sum. No hospital can deliver this much quality care and keep its doors open without significant reimbursement.

The financial aspects of my illness fortunately never became a big issue for me. I've paid high premiums for medical insurance for decades. Throughout that time, insurance companies collected much more from me every year than they paid out. With my heart surgery, this year was different. The bill for my operation and after-care exceeded the total of my previous lifetime medical expenses. The amount was large enough to trigger the catastrophic coverage of my insurance plan. Blue Shield paid my hospital and doctors' charges in full. I did have to shell out for my medications after discharge, which even with insurance co-payment came to several hundred dollars in the first four months after my surgery. I am aware that the same illness causes far more financial hardship for many others and feel fortunate to have avoided that stress.

My biggest financial hit from my illness came from loss of income. Although I had disability insurance, payments from it would have started only after six months. Returning to work in less than half that time, I didn't receive a dime from my policy and missed out on 12 weeks of earnings.

One of my colleagues recently expressed surprise that I returned to work so soon; that I returned to work at all. If I had not, my disability insurance would have kicked in and provided me with adequate income. The stress of being a doctor can be too much for someone with coronary artery disease. Many others have retired after the surgery I had. The thought never even entered my mind. I valued my relationships with patients and colleagues too much. My goal was to get back to normal from the start. I had no plan B.

As William Osler observed, knowing what sort of person has a disease is more important than knowing what disease a patient has. Doctors knew what injuries my gymnastics teammates had, but they underestimated their capacity and motivation to get back to competition in record time. Some patients see an illness as a reason, perhaps as a convenient excuse, to stop working. That can be a smart or a not-so-smart decision. Work provides plenty of rewards besides income. A person who has always longed to do something else may take the opportunity to embark on a different career path after recovery. For those who love and appreciate their jobs and can recuperate enough to continue, returning to their job full-time is the obvious goal. The nature of the person who has the disease often determines the eventual outcome. For me, recovery meant getting back to work, getting back to the life I had before my surgery.

Chapter 17

From Surreality to Reality:
Coming to Terms with Your New Self

Things turn out best for folks who make the
best of the way things turn out.

—attributed to Abraham Lincoln,
John Wooden, and others

A major operation, like any traumatic event fades into
the distance but never quite goes away. Its impact
depends on the severity and duration of the trauma
suffered.

The experience of my illness continues to feel surreal, as if it had happened to someone else. I had been
in robust health nearly all my life and enjoy the same
happy state today. After a bizarre episode that lasted a
few months, I looked several years older. My appearance
played catch-up with the aging process, not completely
but enough to be noticeable. My hairline retreated a bit;
new wrinkles emerged on my face. None of those developments limit how I feel or what I can do. I have a bounce
in my steps again and have to remind myself to slow down
when walking with others.

My life continues as if I had never suffered from coronary artery disease—mainly. The happy-face scar on my
torso has faded from red to pink and finally to a few pale

thin lines. You have to look closely to see the central scar over my sternum. The drain sites have also blanched to white but remain more visible, lingering like the smile of the Cheshire cat. I have normal skin sensation with no residual numbness. With no more tenderness over my chest, I can freely hug others again.

Even my right cephalic vein, the one on the inside of my elbow that appeared to be destroyed by phlebitis, has apparently reincarnated. It may be the same channel or perhaps another that has dilated to take the place of the original. Either way, the vein is large enough to allow taking blood samples with ease.

Nine months after my surgery, Rachel and I moved into a house in Beverly Hills, about a mile from our Century City condo. Ten months after that, Rachel gave birth to our daughter, Kelsee Anne (initials KAK, sounds like cake, our little baby cake). We didn't change any of our plans; my surgery merely delayed some items on our to-do list by a few months. Like many other patients, I have benefitted greatly from my surgery.

That's the view on the surface. Digging a little deeper, however, the picture can turn a bit murkier.

Longevity with good health runs in my family. Born in 1906, when life expectancy was around 47 years, my father lived twice as long, past his 94th birthday. My maternal grandfather, born in the latter years of the nineteenth century, remained active and sharp into his late 80s. With that and my own record of sterling health, I had always expected to live handily beyond the average life span. Since my heart surgery, I am not so sure.

My father lived through very different life events. The maxim that "heredity loads the gun and environment pulls the trigger" may help explain why my heart needed help at an age when my father saw doctors only for routine checkups. What factors in the environment? I wish I knew. Research on that is ongoing and of interest to all of us.

However, my father also benefited from medical intervention. In his mid-70s, he underwent a partial colon resection for cancer but required no additional treatment for a complete cure. In earlier times, that cancer might have shortened his life by over a decade and led to a more painful death.

I hope my operation and subsequent treatment will produce a similar benefit. The results from a coronary artery bypass, particularly those utilizing internal thoracic arteries, are quite good. Over 90 percent of patients are alive ten years after surgery, and the bypass vessels usually remain wide open.[1] Follow-up reports beyond that are fewer in number, since the longer you need to keep track of a group of patients, the more difficult it becomes. One study found that over 60 percent of patients didn't require another intervention in the 18 years following their bypass with an internal thoracic artery.[2] So, with the aid of state-of-the-art medicine, my DNA mixture may yet prove resilient after all.

According to the Center for Disease Control, a white male aged 65 in 2010 (the year I turned 62) had a life expectancy of 18 more years, until he reached age 83.[3] But I have fewer hereditary and lifestyle risk factors than average. On the negative side, I've already suffered the effects of coronary artery disease. My optimism, filtered through a touch of realism, leads me to believe that the odds are in my favor for a longer-than-average stretch. Of course, that's exactly the type of reasoning that made me think I was protected from heart disease—before being proven so very wrong.

Years before my surgery, when my cholesterol first registered at a number high enough to treat, I resisted starting medication. I argued with my doctor and myself, "Taking a statin is beneficial for most people with high cholesterol, but the data wasn't collected on men like me with a great family history and low blood pressure. I work out, have never smoked and am not overweight. How do we know that the benefits outweigh the risks in someone like me?"

For about five years, I tried an alternative strategy—a lower fat diet and hope. When that failed to produce the desired result, I started taking a statin and lowered my cholesterol level to the recommended range. By the time my heart symptoms started, my cholesterol had been under good control for over seven years.

We've all made decisions that may have adversely affected our health. When an illness hits, it's normal to question what we might have done differently to avoid getting sick. I've examined and reexamined my medical history in agonizing detail, searching for what I might have done differently if able to turn back the clock. The best I can come up with is starting on a statin sooner. That may have made a difference, since lower levels of cholesterol in my bloodstream would have meant less cholesterol available to colonize the inside of my coronary arteries. In retrospect, the strategy of trying to reduce my serum cholesterol with dietary changes alone should have been stopped after a few months. But I acted under the illusion that my risk for coronary artery disease was low. Therefore, my desire to avoid taking medication, and to steer clear of its possible side effects, outweighed the potential threat posed by elevated lipids.

Like all powerful drugs, statins can cause harm as well as benefit. They reduce the production of cholesterol in the liver, the desired effect. However, statins can also interfere with other chemical processes and damage liver cells. Consequently, liver function must be monitored periodically with blood tests. The most common statin side effect is muscle pain and weakness. Blood sugar may also increase, and some people develop type 2 diabetes. Before initiating statin therapy, the potential benefit must be evaluated against the potential harm on an individual basis. Treatment can also be modified later, since people may have a problem with one statin drug but not with another. When I felt my heart risk was low, I didn't want to take on the dangers of the side effects of medication, nor the burden of the need to monitor for them. (My assessment was based on the state of medical knowledge then. In the interim, the risks of statins have been reevaluated and found to be significantly lower. If faced with the same situation today, I likely would have started treatment far sooner.)

After my surgery, I didn't need to be talked into taking medicines to reduce my cholesterol even further, to the lower range recommended for people who have already suffered coronary artery disease. Nothing like heart surgery to convince a patient of the need for vigilance. I surely don't want a repeat experience—with its risks, pain, complications, and disruption of life. Fortunately, I've escaped all the harmful statin side effects, at least so far.

Some people believe in fate, that our destiny is predetermined before we are born. I emphatically do not. How we act can improve or diminish our future. The evidence for that is overwhelming. My parents changed my family's destiny by moving to the other side of the world, from Europe to America, for a better life. Each of us has the opportunity to walk or run in the cross-country race of life. The results of our decisions are enormously consequential. Fate can be fickle, but people who practice healthy habits, monitor their well-being and take advantage of medical treatments improve their prospects for a longer, more active life. The motto of the American Society of Anesthesiologists is a single word, "Vigilance." I practice that in safeguarding the health of my patients and my own.

My biggest revelation from heart surgery is that my time on this earth is finite. Of course I knew that before—I just never felt it. Having been hit over the head with a proverbial brick, I am no longer oblivious to this fundamental existential reality. In the immediate aftermath of my operation, I focused totally on recovering my usual state of vigorous health. I didn't think about the more distant future. After I got back to my normal self and had additional time to reflect, some doubt started creeping in. It didn't happen right away, and it doesn't dominate my thinking, but an uneasy feeling about my vulnerability pops up intermittently. When I come down with a bad cold or indigestion, particularly if I feel a slight discomfort anywhere near my chest, I inevitably wonder whether it's the harbinger of something more ominous.

Doctors, patients, and even philosophers describe our attempts to recover from illness with the language of war. We battle an illness, defeat a disease. That can accurately describe an acute episode, like the blockages treated with my surgery, but not the challenges posed by a chronic and progressive process. My coronary artery disease revealed a tendency to form atherosclerotic deposits, which can compromise circulation in any artery throughout my body. Heart surgery solved the immediate problem but didn't eliminate the lifetime risk posed by atherosclerosis. That includes damage from coatings of fat, calcium, and other debris already deposited in arteries throughout my body and additional layers that are likely to accumulate, including in the bypass vessels in my heart. I plan to do everything possible to reduce the progression of this process—with drugs, diet, and exercise—but this is a chronic illness that I have to live with, not something I can defeat once and forget.

I have been particularly concerned about decreased endurance during vigorous exercise. Dr. Drury chalks it up to advancing years, and he is almost surely right. The beta blocker I take can also cause decreased exercise capacity, and tweaking my dose or changing to a different medicine might help.

I feel good. I feel strong. I have no limitations on my physical activity. But given my history, it's hard to shake nagging doubts about what the future might hold. Having been ambushed by illness once, I am more acutely aware that such unpleasant surprises are part of the danger we all face.

The necessity of having to undergo heart surgery also wounded me psychologically. My heart is scarred, metaphorically as well as physically. I will never again be able to imagine myself a lucky recipient of exceptional good health. Previously, that had been a bedrock of my identity. I can never fully shed the stigma of being a heart patient.

It's a negative part of my résumé. Nobody wants to be a heart patient.

I don't fear death itself. What I dread is not living long enough to do all the things I had envisioned myself doing. Some people call this a "bucket list." I've never made such a list; I don't think I could ever empty the bucket. Just as soon as one item is crossed off the list, new goals spontaneously pop up to take its place. But I expected to live long enough to travel to many more marvelous places, to write several books, and to see my daughter grow up. I still think I'll get to do all those things, but a delayed-onset aftereffect of my surgery is that doubt has crept in.

Maybe I need to travel to remote places like Papua New Guinea and Lake Titicaca sooner, to dodge the risk that health issues might prevent me from doing so later. I feel a greater urgency to get more words down on paper or computer screen before time runs out on finishing the books I want to write.

There is always more, no matter what goals you reach, no matter what triumphs you achieve. The city champion in any sport longs to win the state and then the national title; the national champ strives to win the world crown. Even those talented and fortunate enough to achieve such a lofty prize soon desire even higher acclaim, such as "the greatest of all time."

Distinguished university commencement speakers sometimes tell new graduates that nobody ever wished on their deathbed that they had spent more time at the office. While that may be true, it's totally misleading because of the focus on the mundane instead of the satisfaction that comes from accomplishment. Plenty of people wish they had enjoyed greater success in their careers, achieved more, produced a richer legacy, a greater lasting positive impact on their community and society at large. That may at times require devoting more energy to your career, and yes, spending more time at the office.

The question comes down to how to live life with the most meaning. Each of us faces the challenge of how to best balance our time between personal obligations and responsibilities to society at large. Devoting more time to work often takes away from personal relationships and vice versa. Living well demands an agile balancing act. Many people feel guilty about slighting both their work and their family, maybe even at the same time. The sad and happy reality is that there are more worthwhile things to do than hours in a day.

After a life-threatening illness, people tend to reexamine their priorities and life goals. Some choose to retire from their careers, concentrate on maintaining their health and enriching personal relationships. Depending on circumstances, including age and level of recovery, that can be a reasonable decision.

Other people refocus on different goals. Some change from a corporate job to one in public service or the arts. I plan to focus more on my writing, to better fulfill an artistic desire and hopefully make a positive contribution to my readers. My medical career made it difficult for me to devote enough time and effort to writing in the past. But it's certainly possible to fashion such a dual career. Many physicians have managed to produce important books.

I don't like to think of myself as a heart patient, as any kind of patient. I use all my medical know-how to rationalize that I am not as sick as others with a similar medical history. What I want to feel, how I actually do feel, contradicts what I know intellectually. I try to ignore this dissonance but can't help being aware of it.

"That which does not kill us," Friedrich Nietzsche claimed, "makes us stronger." He couldn't be more wrong when it comes to illness. Plenty of people survive a medical crisis and come out weaker for the experience. It could be a stroke, the loss of a limb, a heart attack, or numerous other maladies that leave the patient diminished. I don't have a physical limitation from my illness, but doubt has crept in where previously only confidence dwelled. So, despite all my protestations, I do see myself as a heart patient, at least some of the time. The disease hangs over me, not as ominously as the sword of Damocles, but present just the same.

I don't often dwell on this. I'm usually too busy fulfilling obligations, making plans, enjoying hobbies, entertainment, and the companionship of family and friends—you know, living. But during my recuperation, I had ample time to reflect on some core issues that on ordinary days don't demand urgent attention—the all-important question of "What have you done with your life?" and, even more significant, "What do you plan to do with the rest of it?"

As noted, illness is a family affair. A major operation almost inevitably alters a patient's life, sense of self, and narrative for the future. It inspires reflection and efforts for positive changes. All this affects the patient's family as well. Reassessment can be contagious.

Besides me, the person most profoundly affected by my surgery shared every day of it. The experience changed Rachel's life as well. This next section is Rachel's account.

Prior to his illness, Andrew had been so strong, so full of energy. Seeing him in the ICU right after surgery, looking so vulnerable, was a shock. It made me realize on a gut level just how fragile life is.

During my drive home the night after the surgery, I felt so alone. Prior to my marriage, I had lived alone for many years and never felt lonely. But after finding love with the man I wanted to spend my life with, it was different. I felt so very lonely in our apartment all by myself. Our bed felt empty and cold without Andrew. I knew I didn't want my life to be that way. That bolstered my already strong determination to make sure Andrew recovered.

Another thing that changed was my approach to arguments. I am pretty strongheaded and was used to winning arguments. My usual modus operandi was to press my point of view as long as it took to prevail. As Andrew was recuperating, I realized that my relationship with him was more important to me than

any argument. That's when I decided that whenever
I started getting mad, I would ask for a time-out to
avoid saying something hurtful I would later regret. I
still maintain my position as long as I feel I'm right, but
I think more about the other person's feelings. I don't
want the heat of the moment to burn a permanent
injury. I think living through this experience has made
me more mellow and tolerant.

While I was single, I didn't do much cooking.
I'd make simple meals for myself or eat out. During
Andrew's recuperation, I decided to prepare comfort foods for him. That led me to YouTube videos of
Hungarian cooking. Andrew now calls me the best
Hungarian cook in Beverly Hills. I did have the starting advantage of inheriting a kitchenful of cooking
supplies, pots, and dishes from Andrew's mother,
whom everyone considered an outstanding cook. I
wish she had been around to teach me. Andrew was
no help. He told me, "My specialty is eating, not
cooking." He was, however, always encouraging.
The worst he would tell me was that a meal was
good but not exactly the way the traditional version
tasted. After a few attempts, I was able to prepare
wiener schnitzel, chicken paprikash, and *palacsinta*
(crepes) like a pro.

Before Andrew's illness, we were both very busy
with our careers. While he was home recuperating,
we had an opportunity to spend more time together.
I felt closer to him. We went from newlyweds to a
family. I felt loved and appreciated. Sometimes I still
miss having so much time alone together.

I wrote this book primarily for people facing surgery, long-term illness, or hospitalization and for their loved ones. I wanted to provide hope for those confronting a difficult and painful recovery, and to describe some medical procedures, the rationale behind them, and the process of recuperation. Knowing what's going on can make it easier for patients to understand and accept what they need to do to help themselves heal. And seeing that others have traveled down the same road with good results can be encouraging.

A note of caution here: you or your loved one will not face the same sequence of complications and challenges, nor the same path to recovery that I went through. However, I believe that there will be enough similarities to make my story informative and helpful.

If you're facing surgery, you're bound to feel anxious. Please do keep in mind that the vast majority of patients recover well. If anybody tells you that you won't suffer any pain after a major operation, don't believe them. When patients ask me if they will have pain after surgery, my usual answer is, "Yes, but you'll have pain medication available whenever you need it." As a wound heals, the pain diminishes. You may have some setbacks or complications. They will most likely respond to treatment. Your life will be turned upside down—by sleep disturbance, night sweats, and other symptoms that will go away within days or weeks. After a few months, you'll most likely be able to return to your usual activities. For individual concerns, do consult your own doctors.

During the writing of this book, I was reminded that much of what happens in heart disease applies to other major illnesses. The lessons I learned could have wider application to anyone facing a medical crisis and their loved ones. That includes just about anybody, at least for some portions of their lives.

The chaplain at Cedars-Sinai once gave a sermon on the biblical imperative to "be a blessing." He saw this as a commandment to enrich the lives of people we know and touch by supporting their goals and dreams. During my time-out of usual life due to illness, I thought about what paying more attention to that directive could accomplish. I believe that I've had a net positive impact on people I've met in life. At least I hope that's true. But I also feel the angst voiced by the fictitious Private Ryan at the gravesite of the man who saved him. "Have I lived a good life?" he asked. In my case, have I lived a life worthy of the struggles and sacrifices made by my parents and their ancestors, this country's founders, and countless others whose "blood, toil, tears, and sweat" created the relatively comfortable world I inherited?

I could have taken time out for similar reflection without heart surgery. Anyone can at any time. But as Samuel Johnson noted centuries ago, a dramatic event forces the issue and concentrates the mind.

Until my illness, I lived as if my time on this earth had no endpoint. My heart disease has forced me to evaluate decisions with an awareness that my time is finite. I regret that I lacked the wisdom to do so decades ago.

I am most fortunate to be living in a time when medical science has already developed an effective treatment for my manifestation of coronary artery disease. In all likelihood at some future date the treatment for this condition will be far easier, sparing patients from the difficult recuperation I went through. A "minimally invasive" version of the coronary artery bypass operation, one that eliminates splitting of the breastbone by making a two-to-three-inch incision between two ribs and a couple of additional holes for the insertion of instruments, has already been introduced. Unfortunately, such an approach was not the appropriate one to repair my pathology. But had I been born just a few decades earlier, I would have faced the prospect of severe restrictions on my activities, constrained by chest pain and the constant threat of sudden death. I would have had to stop working. Travel to remote places would have posed too high a risk. So, I continue to be grateful for my good fortune, not just in enjoying good health but for all the other opportunities I've had and continue to have for a happy and fulfilling life.

Since my heart surgery, I think more about how I spend my time and how what I do impacts others. I compliment people more often, to make sure they know that their good deeds elicit appreciation and gratitude. I am more focused and determined to make a positive impact on my family, friends, and community. As a result, at least in some ways, this difficult interlude has also made my life better.

Patients can emerge from a major illness and live the rest of their lives with a better perspective on what's important to them. As with any trial, people can become scarred for life or more empowered to live their best lives. Often the outcome is both. If you are facing a major surgery, you can take heart in knowing that you can live a happy and satisfying life for a long time afterward.

Epilogue

You live it [life] forward, but understand it
backward.

—Abraham Verghese

More than a dozen years have passed since I completed the original draft of this book. In the interim,
my life has continued mostly as it would have if I never
had heart surgery. I continue to take medicines to prevent
recurrence (or at least delay) of heart problems and get
periodic checkups. Fortunately, I've had no symptoms of
heart disease since my recuperation.

I continued working at Cedars-Sinai for a dozen years
after my heart surgery. In 2022, at age 74 and 46 years
after doing my first case at Cedars, I joined the emeritus
staff, doctors who no longer treat patients. That has given
me more time to polish this book for publication and to
write articles.

Kelsee is now a thriving sixth grader. Rachel and I
have already visited Taiwan and Hungary with her.
Together we've hiked in Yosemite, Zion, and Bryce Can-
yon National Parks. Yellowstone and lots of other magnificent locations remain on our travel wish list. I have
had the opportunity to tour both Lake Titicaca and Papua

New Guinea. In 2023, I trekked at 7,000-feet altitude to see mountain gorillas scampering in their forest home in Rwanda.

An active life is not only possible but quite likely after heart surgery and many other major illnesses. My hope is that readers of this book will be encouraged by knowing that.

Acknowledgments

I present this chronicle as a thank-you note to all the people who helped me through this process: my family, friends, doctors, nurses, therapists, and other hospital personnel. I am most grateful for the kind gestures and good wishes of friends and coworkers, many of whom went out of their way to show their support with words and thoughtful gifts. Having been on the receiving end, I have an even stronger appreciation for the quality of care provided by Cedars-Sinai and feel prouder than ever to be part of that care for others.

I want to acknowledge, in particular, the kind and capable treatment provided by my cardiologist, Dr. Kevin Drury; surgeon, Dr. Alfredo Trento; and anesthesiologist, Dr. Nicola D'Attellis. I have mentioned throughout the text a number of other doctors, nurses, and therapists who also played important roles in my recuperation. A big thank-you and a heartfelt standing ovation to each and every one of you.

Producing a book is a collaborative effort and I want to recognize and thank some of the people who played significant roles in getting this project across the finish line. Eric Lincoln Miller of 3ibooks Literary Agency worked diligently to find my publisher and expertly guided the book through the publishing process. Philip Marino and

Laurie Harting, my editors at Morehouse Publishing, skillfully chaperoned the project through its final phase. I am grateful to all the people who gave me feedback and helped edit my writing along the way. Deanna Brady was especially helpful with encouraging and expert advice.

I particularly want to thank two stalwart members of my three-person writing group, Deborah Dahan and Bruce Gale, for their friendship and all the helpful feedback they have given me over the years. I also want to thank my writing teachers: professors in the UCLA Extension Writing Program—particularly Linda Marsa, David Ulin, and Susan Vaughn; and, in the Antioch University Creative Writing MFA program, particularly Peter Selgin and Sharman Apt Russell.

I also wish to thank Dr. James Forrester, distinguished cardiologist and author, for his support and encouragement.

I want to express my deep gratitude to family members who provided love and support throughout my illness: Christine Gregory, Kenny Kadar, and especially Rachel, my wife, who provided amazing help to me every step of the way.

Notes

Chapter 1: Recognizing the Unseen:
The Subtlety of Symptoms

1. Harvard Medical School Heart Health Newsletter, November 3, 2020; Véronique L. Roger et al., "Heart Disease and Stroke Statistics—2011 Update: A Report From the American Heart Association, *Circulation* 123, no. 4 (2011), e18–e209, doi:10.1161/CIR.0b013e3182009701; and J. R. Margolis et al., "Eighteen-Year Follow-Up: The Framingham Study," *The American Journal of Cardiology* 32, no. 1 (1973), 1–7, doi:10.1016/s0002-9149(73)80079-7.

2. Z. J. Zheng et al., "Sudden Cardiac Death in the United States, 1989 to 1998," *Circulation* 104, no. 18 (2001), 2158–63, doi:10.1161/hc4301.098254; and James Forrester, *The Heart Healers: The Misfits, Mavericks, and Rebels Who Created the Greatest Medical Breakthrough of Our Lives* (New York: St. Martin's Press, 2015), 1.

Chapter 3: Embracing Your New Reality:
The Power of Acceptance

1. Mayo Clinic Staff, "Positive Thinking: Stop Negative Self-talk to Reduce Stress," mayoclinic.org, Mayo Clinic, November 21, 2023, https://www.mayoclinic.org/healthy-lifestyle/stress-management/in-depth/positive-thinking/art-20043950, accessed December 3, 2023.

2. Karen Feldscher, "How the Power of Positive Thinking Works," *Harvard Gazette*, December 7, 2016, https://news.harvard.edu/gazette/story/2016/12/optistic-women-live-longer-are

-healthier/, accessed December 3, 2023; summarizing from Eric S. Kim et al., "Optimism and Cause-Specific Mortality: A Prospective Cohort Study," Harvard T. H. Chan School of Public Health, *American Journal of Epidemiology* 185, no. 1 (2017), 21–29, https://doi.org/10.1093/aje/kww182.

3. Martin S. Hagger, Severine Koch, Nikos L. D. Chatzisarantis, and Sheina Orbell, "The Common Sense Model of Self-Regulation: Meta-Analysis and Test of a Process Model," *Psychological Bulletin* 143, no. 11 (2017), 1117–54, https://doi.org/10.1037/bul0000118, accessed December 3, 2023.

4. Yasmine Phillips, "Research Shows Positive or Negative Attitude Impacts Illness Recovery," curtin.edu, Curtin University, August 16, 2017, https://www.curtin.edu.au/news/media-release/research-shows-positive-negative-attitude-impacts-illness-recovery/, accessed December 3, 2023.

Chapter 4: Turning Points:
Surgery and the Miracles of Modern Medicine

1. Susannah Fox, "Friends, Family & Post-surgical Outcomes," pewresearch.org, Pew Research Center, February 20, 2008, https://www.pewresearch.org/internet/2008/02/20/friends-family-post-surgical-outcomes/#:~:text=Surgical%20patients%20with%20a%20strong,%2Dsurgical%20follow%2Dup%20days, accessed December 3, 2023.

Chapter 5: Awakening: The Dawn of Recovery

1. Khadije Daneshjou et al., "Congenital Insensitivity to Pain and Anhydrosis (CIPA) Syndrome; A Report of 4 Cases," *Iranian Journal of Pediatrics* 22, no. 3 (2012), 412–6.

Chapter 8: Perseverance Through Pain:
The Marathon of Healing

1. American Psychological Association, "Perseverance Toward Life Goals Can Fend Off Depression, Anxiety, Panic Disorders," apa.org, American Psychological Association, May 2,

2019, https://www.apa.org/news/press/releases/2019/05/goals
-perseverance, accessed December 3, 2023.

Chapter 11: Seeking Equilibrium:
Finding Balance in the Extremes

1. Waguih William IsHak et al., "Screening for Depression in
Hospitalized Medical Patients," *Journal of Hospital Medicine* 12,
no. 2 (2017), 118–25, doi:10.12788/jhm.2693, accessed December 3, 2023.

Chapter 14: Reflections: A Shift in Perspectives

1. "Health Benefits of Gratitude," uclahealth.org, UCLA Health,
March 2, 2023, https://www.uclahealth.org/news/health
-benefits-gratitude, accessed December 3, 2023.

Chapter 17: From Surreality to Reality:
Coming to Terms with Your New Self

1. F. D. Loop et al., "Influence of the Internal-Mammary-Artery
Graft on 10-Year Survival and Other Cardiac Events," *The New
England Journal of Medicine* 314, no. 1 (1986), 1–6, doi:10.1056
/NEJM198601023140101.
2. M. J. Boylan et al., "Surgical Treatment of Isolated Left Anterior Descending Coronary Stenosis. Comparison of Left Internal
Mammary Artery and Venous Autograft at 18 to 20 Years of
Follow-Up," *The Journal of Thoracic and Cardiovascular Surgery*
107, no. 3 (1994), 657–62.
3. Elizabeth Arias, United States Life Tables, 2010. National
Vital Statistics Reports, CDC, p.3, Table A.